344 10441
BYRNE

Rights & Wrongs in M

LIVERPOOL LIBRARIES AND ARTS

DATE DUE FOR RETURN

16 DEC 1987

13 1.

11 JUL 1988

22.3 91

7 DEC 1988

25 JAN 1989

20 FEB 1989

31 JUL 1989

1 - MAR 1991

X

Books may be renewed by personal call, telephone or post.

COMMERCIAL LIBRARY

R 267

Rights and Wrongs in Medicine:
King's College Studies 1985–6

Rights and Wrongs in Medicine
King's College Studies 1985–6

Edited by Peter Byrne

King Edward's Hospital Fund for London

© King Edward's Hospital Fund for London 1986

Printed and bound in England
by Oxford University Press

Distributed for the King's Fund by Oxford University Press

ISBN 0 19 724637 0

King's Fund Publishing Office
2 St Andrew's Place
London NW1 4LB

CONTENTS

Preface Peter Byrne	6
A survey of the year 1. The doctor–patient relationship Ian Kennedy	7
A survey of the year 2. The limits of medical advance Peter Byrne	22
Re-reading Warnock Simon Lee	37
Persons, kinds and capacities Keith Ward	53
Warnock and surrogate motherhood: sentiment or argument? Shelley Roberts	80
The Jewish contribution to medical ethics Sir Immanuel Jakobovits	115
Unemployment and health Stephen Farrow	127
Responsibility: law, medicine or morals? Nicola Lacey	139
Parents, children and medical treatment: the legal issues Brenda Hoggett	158
Everyday ethics: prevention, paternalism and the pill Roger Higgs	177
Index	194

PREFACE

The Centre of Medical Law and Ethics at King's College London was founded in 1978 to provide opportunities for teaching, study, research and discussion of issues in medicine which involve consideration of law and ethics. From its inception the Centre has taken as its aim to encourage the investigation of matters, both theoretical and practical, transcending the frontiers of medicine, law and ethics. An annual series of public lectures in medical law and ethics has been one of the major instruments in trying to achieve this aim.

The Centre now offers these lectures for publication for the first time, together with a number of invited papers of related interest. The contributors are drawn from a wide range of disciplines and represent diverse interests. There has been no attempt by the editor to tailor their views to fit a party line. Each has been allowed to speak freely.

It is planned that this will be the first in an annual series of volumes on medical law and ethics. Each will begin with 'A Survey of the Year' reviewing the important developments in medical law and ethics of the preceding twelve months. The remaining essays will naturally also tend to reflect those issues that have been in the forefront of recent controversy: hence the concentration in the present volume upon matters relating to artifically assisted reproduction and to the Gillick judgement.

We hope that what is offered in these pages will stimulate reflection and debate on the ethical and legal issues that surround contemporary medical practice and will inaugurate a series that will come to be viewed as an important source of comment on these issues.

Peter Byrne

A SURVEY OF THE YEAR
1. THE DOCTOR–PATIENT RELATIONSHIP
Ian Kennedy

Until relatively recently, medical law referred, if it referred to anything, to medical malpractice, that area of law concerned with doctors' negligence. Significant, even dramatic, developments may have taken place in medical practice. There was, however, little or no parallel development in the law. Special problems were not met with special legal solutions, although they undoubtedly raised legal issues of great complexity. Consider developments in reproductive medicine, contraception, transplants, genetic counselling, the care of the new-born, the use of intensive care and research on human subjects (including, or not, as the argument takes you, human embryos). It cannot be doubted that the law quite properly has something to say about each of these. Equally it cannot be doubted that the law has been exceedingly slow or reluctant (or both) to speak up.

Explanations for this are not hard to find. There are two ways in which we make new law or develop the existing law. One is by legislation, the other is through judicial decisions, as a consequence of litigation. It cannot come as any surprise that Parliament, when faced with such enormously taxing issues as the lawfulness of selective treatment of new-born babies, or put more bluntly, letting some babies die, has not exactly jumped at the chance to set the law straight. There are no votes to be won, only to be lost. Politicians, as a consequence, have, by and large, kept their heads down and run for cover or, at best called for the appointment of a commission or committee, that well known parliamentary delaying tactic.

The courts, equally, have had little opportunity to act, even if they were willing to do so. Judicial law-making depends on cases being brought and, until recently, the cost, time and effort of litigation was just too much trouble to be worth it, particularly if the result was, necessarily, extremely hard to predict. Furthermore, judge-made law is not a particularly good way of proceeding. It tends to be interstitial, limited to its facts and, in any case, judges can rarely be persuaded to paint with a broad brush when the pencil or the crayon will do nicely to fill in the particular gap.

A further and, perhaps, more fundamental reason for the undeveloped nature of medical law, has been the conviction held by many, not least those practising medicine, that the law in truth is not involved. They mean, of course, that they do not wish it to be involved. And they have been quite successful in persuading others. Their conviction grows out of two propositions, both wholly untenable. The first is that anything to do with medicine, by virtue of its being 'medical', is best left to the medical profession since they are the experts. The same argument has been used as regards medical ethics, though I doubt if it would be as strongly held if business ethics were being discussed and the view was put forward that the adjective 'business' entailed that it was a matter only for businessmen. Such a view would produce one of the shortest books ever written! The second proposition is that the law really has no place in regulating medicine, that it is too clumsy a tool, too blunt an instrument for the subtleties and complexities of medicine and the doctor–patient relationship. But this is simply (or not so simply) to misunderstand both the nature of law and its applicability to medicine. Law is not necessarily clumsy, nor is it necessarily over-restrictive (nor, that other cliché, rigid). It can be sensitive to the needs of the doctor and patient. After all, the general legal principle governing the conduct of doctors is only that they behave as reasonable doctors, a question to be resolved by medical evidence. Furthermore, law cannot be kept out of the consulting room or surgery. It is there already. Whenever someone lays hands on another, and, *a fortiori*, takes a knife to his flesh, society takes it sufficiently seriously that it looks to its most formal method of social ordering, the law, to make sure the line is held between the tolerable and the intolerable.

So, in short, the law should have plenty to say about modern medical developments but, for a variety of reasons, has been disturbingly silent.

I say 'has been' because, over the last five years or so, things have slowly begun to change. The growing realisation that the law is involved, but is far from clear, has resulted in an increasing number of cases being brought before the courts.

The courts have been the focus of activity, *faute de mieux*, since, as has been seen, Parliament would prefer, apparently, not to be involved. The drawbacks of judicial law making have been accepted in the spirit of better some guide to conduct rather than none at all, particularly if there is otherwise the threat that someone, somewhere could also bring a lawsuit or, worse, a prosecution to challenge what had been thought previously to be good practice.

Thus, besides a gradual increase in malpractice cases, there have been cases concerned with abortion, *Royal College of Nursing v DHSS* [1981] AC 800; consent, *Sidaway v Board of Governors of the Bethlem Royal Hospital and the Maudsley Hospital* [1985] 2 WLR 480; the selective treatment of new-born babies, *In re B* (a minor) [1981] 1 WLR 1421 and *R v Arthur (1981) 283, British Medical Journal*; 'wrongful life', *McKay v Essex Area Health Authority* [1982] 2 All ER 771; the prescription of contraceptives to young girls, *Gillick v West Norfolk and Wisbech Area Health Authority* [1985] 1 All ER 533; failed sterilisation operations, *Emeh v Kensington and Chelsea and Westminster Area Health Authority* [1984] 3 All ER 1044; and legal action is pending over the use of the drug Opren and the whooping cough vaccine.

It is important to seek an explanation for this recent flurry of litigation, which will probably increase in intensity over the next few years. There are probably two levels of explanation. The first, more superficial level, involves the need, more or less urgent, to clarify the law where daily conduct may suddenly be brought into question. The deeper level, however, is perhaps the more interesting one. For this litigation should be understood as representing part of a continuing process of defining and redefining the doctor–patient relationship.

There are, of course, many ways, formal and informal, in which this relationship is constantly reshaped. How a doctor perceives and regards a patient, and the patient a doctor, is the consequence of a whole set of complicated social assumptions and conventions. And it has already been seen that some, especially some doctors, would prefer the nature of the relationship to be shaped only by the ebb and flow of social custom and cultural values. But there are others who see this as an unsatisfactory method of writing the rules for the relationship. They argue that the power of the professional, since he is the one with the knowledge and skills whom the patient approaches for help, means that if informal social mechanisms are relied upon, there will never be any real departure from the parent–child relationship which they claim has characterised the doctor–patient relationship for decades. This is because informal social mechanisms reflect necessarily the existing pattern of social forces. Thus if the doctor is the figure with power, he is likely to remain so, and any reshaping of his relationship with the patient will be subject to this overriding constraint. This has persuaded some people to have recourse to the formal social mechanism of the law by inviting the court to set the terms of the relationship.

Putting it another way, the gradual and increasing growth in recourse to litigation stems from two basic premises. The first is a dissatisfaction with, and a desire to depart from, the prevailing relationship in which the doctor is a dominant father-figure whose views should prevail not just on diagnosis, prognosis and treatment, the world of medical technique, but also on what the doctor and the patient ought to do, the world of medical ethics and law. They aim at a relationship which is closer to a partnership of equals, in which each party respects the needs and claims of the other.

The second premise is the conviction that such a departure from the existing relationship, such a redefinition of roles, will only be possible by recourse to a system outside the world of medicine and a system which is formal and has authority. The notion that the medical profession will *sua sponte* take on a different and, by definition, less powerful role is rejected. The rejection stems not from distrust, nor from any belief in the inevitable conservatism of doctors. Rather, it is the product of a belief that patterns of behaviour which are entrenched can be changed only by pressure from outside. So, recourse is had to the courts. There is, of course, a certain naiveté in this, since the courts are peopled by judges who themselves are fellow-professionals, not easily persuaded of the view that doctor or lawyer does not always know best. It is for this reason that I say recourse is had to the courts, *faute de mieux*, there being no other obvious institution to turn to.

It does not follow, therefore, that going to the courts has produced any particularly significant reshaping of the doctor-patient relationship. The conservatism of the law and the courts, together with the sense of fraternal professionalism, mean that decisions handed down by the courts are as likely to entrench prevailing attitudes as to augur new ones. Nonetheless, it remains my submission that the growth of medical–legal litigation must be understood as part, and a major part, of the social process of defining the proper bounds of the doctor-patient relationship.

Litigation is not, of course, the only or even, perhaps, the most noticeable way in which tensions in the doctor–patient relationship have been and are explored. Revisions in the British Medical Association's *The Handbook of Medical Ethics* and in the General Medical Council's 'Blue Book' (*Professional Conduct and Discipline*) represent efforts by the medical profession and others to take account of and respond to pressure for change. Equally important is the increase in public discussion of medical ethics in particular and the role and status of the professions in general in the press and broadcasts, and the reaction it produces. And, of course, the considerable increase in scholarly writing has had its impact.

With this introduction, it is instructive to refer briefly to some recent developments in medical law as illustrations of what I have called this 'social process'. I shall concentrate initially on two cases which have wound their way through the courts right up to the highest court, the House of Lords. This fact is, in itself, significant, demonstrating the preparedness of parties to settle down to a long fight, taking several years – let alone the cost involved in money, effort and time. You only do this when you take something very seriously, when something important is at stake. What is at stake in these cases, and others which I am sure will follow, is the very nature of the doctor–patient relationship.

Sidaway v Board of Governors of the Bethlem Royal Hospital and the Maudsley Hospital [1985] 2 WLR 480

In this case, Mrs Sidaway underwent an operation on her neck to relieve what had become intractable pain in her arm and shoulder. Sadly, her spinal cord was damaged in the course of the operation and she suffered partial paralysis. Expert evidence was given at the trial that there was a risk of such paralysis, but it was of the order of less than one per cent. Mrs Sidaway was not told of this risk before the operation. She sued the surgeon claiming that she should have been informed. The trial judge found as a fact that she had not been informed of that risk and that, if she had, she would not have agreed to the operation.

What should concern us here is not some lengthy exegesis of the law as stated by the courts at each level. That can be found elsewhere (for example, Grubb, 'Medical Malpractice in England', 1, Journal of Contemporary Health Law and Policy, 75, (1985)). Our question is more general. What bearing on the doctor–patient relationship does the case have? Shortly put, the case concerned consent to treatment. The courts were being asked to set the ground rules under which consent must be sought and given. And although in strict terms they were only asked to adjudicate the dispute between Mrs Sidaway and her doctor, they were being invited to state what the law demands by way of consent. It was an invitation which was readily accepted.

Consent is important, of course, as an issue because it is quintessentially concerned with power. Consent is a feature, or reflection, of autonomy. It gives expression to the notion of self-determination. If a doctor may not treat a patient without that patient's consent, subject, perhaps, to exceptions, each of which needs justification, then a statement is being made that a patient's autonomy is important. And, on this, the law at one level has always been clear. Consent is required. But this is a rather crude proposition. It means that doctors cannot treat by force or trick, but doctors do not do this. The real question is, given that consent is important, how important is it. This resolves into two questions; what is required of the doctor and the patient before consent is real and, parallel with this, who decides. The House of Lords in *Sidaway* decided that it was properly a matter for them to decide. But this still left the other issue; what decision should they make.

The claim was made that consent to be real must *inter alia* be informed. This merely reflects the proposition that you cannot be said to agree to something if you do not know what you are agreeing to. But this leads straight to the centre of the controversy. How much information does the patient have to have, how much is he entitled to know, before it can be said that he knew what he was agreeing to? The answer is crucial in the continuing efforts to shape and reshape the doctor–patient relationship. If the patient's consent can validly be gained by informing him only of those matters, including risks, which the doctor thinks it wise for him to know, then the power to guide the relationship lies with the doctor. Partnership is ousted by paternalism. Undoubtedly, the doctor will do what he does out of a desire to serve the best interests of the patient. But this is merely to state the problem in different terms. For, the question then becomes, who is the better judge of those best interests, the doctor or the patient.

If, on the other hand, consent is only valid if the information to be given is that which the patient makes clear he wishes to know, then a form of partnership is more possible. The doctor, possessed of the skill and the facts, offers his skill and informs the patient of the facts. The patient weighs the facts and then either accepts or refuses the doctor's offer. The doctor remains, if you will, the senior partner, and may, if circumstances warrant, properly decide not to put certain information before the patient if it would trigger a wholly unwarranted and unfortunate response. But, on this approach, the law gives appropriate recognition to the patient's entitlement to know.

Well, these were the arguments before the House of Lords. It will be no surprise that there was no agreement among their Lordships on the general issue, though all agreed, on the particular facts, that Mrs Sidaway's case was not made out. They clearly perceived the case to be of the greatest possible significance in setting the tone and terms of the relationship between doctors and patients for the future. And, I would submit, they gave by their speeches a clear indication that the law was no longer committed to the notion of 'doctor knows best'. They did so cautiously. They did not opt for a rule of law by which each patient was entitled to be informed of all risks and each doctor was under a duty to supply that information. Four of the five Law Lords were not prepared even to go as far as Lord Scarman and adopt what has been called the 'reasonable patient' test; that a patient is entitled to such information as a reasonable patient would wish to know.

Instead, three of their Lordships rejected Lord Diplock's view that a patient need only be told that which a reasonable doctor thought proper to tell, and thereby signalled a gradual movement towards a greater respect for patient autonomy. That they hedged their opinions with caveats should not be allowed to mislead. Nor should the solemn views of those who saw the decisions of the majority of the House as a victory for medical conservatism and paternalism be taken too seriously. Such views are far too pessimistic. The case, properly understood, represents a significant step towards realising the goal of partnership between doctor and patient. The dynamic nature of the law, its capacity to adapt to changed views was again demonstrated. Equally clearly demonstrated was the careful way in which the courts choose to adapt the law. They do it judiciously, giving due warning of the direction it is moving in, careful not to take people too much by surprise, careful not to upset too abruptly established patterns of behaviour.

But, nonetheless, the writing is on the wall. At least as far as consent is concerned, doctors' power unchecked by others, while it should not (quite properly) be replaced by patients' power, is no longer acceptable to the law. Some more equal relationship is what is called for, and this is what will gradually emerge.

That said, any discussion of developments in the law of consent and their implications for the doctor–patient relationship, should not overlook the case of *Freeman v Home Office* [1984] 1 All ER 1036. In that case, a prisoner in jail argued that he was given treatment against his will. The larger issue before the court was the anomalous position of the prison doctor (and any other such doctor-employee), who was employed by the prison service and, therefore, obliged to serve its needs, but, at the same time, was doctor to the prisoner and obliged to serve his needs.

Any alleged consent by a prisoner in such cases, Freeman

argued, was inevitably tainted by coercion and was invalid. It was not, he urged, given voluntarily but under duress, the duress being that the doctor, as a prison officer, had disciplinary functions and was also obliged to report to the prison governor information acquired during consultations which could affect the running of the prison.

Clearly, the court here was being asked to decide something more than the narrow issue of consent. They were being asked to decide that when a doctor has a conflict of loyalties, the *increased* power this gives him, because he must report back to his employer and the patient knows this but cannot prevent it, means that he is disqualified from acting as a doctor, from entering into the relationship of doctor and patient, unless the patient agrees to the arrangement at the outset. In the event, the court rejected this view, although they said that careful attention should be paid to possible conflicts of interest. It is doubtful, however, whether this is the last word on what is a vitally important issue of freedom and power as they affect and condition the doctor–patient relationship.

Gillick v West Norfolk and Wisbech Area Health Authority [1985] 1 All ER 533

This case raises a host of legal issues touching on the practice of medicine. This is not the place to explore it in detail; it is extensively discussed in Brenda Hoggett's essay. Its importance here for me and, indeed, its central importance as a case, lies in the deceptively simple question: when can a person be a patient so as to receive treatment from a doctor? Put another way, what is required for a relationship of doctor and patient to come into being? You may wish to keep this question always in mind as you read Mrs Hoggett's paper.

Mrs Gillick sought a declaration from the court that the Secretary of State acted unlawfully when he advised doctors and health authorities that, in exceptional cases, girls below the age of 16 may be given contraceptive treatment without their parents' knowledge or consent.

Mrs Gillick invited the court (finally, the House of Lords) to resolve a social issue of great contemporary importance and controversy, the nature in law of the relationship between parent and child. By choosing to do so in the context of medical practice, she was also, necessarily, inviting the court to shape the doctor–patient relationship. And the shape she argued for is one which does not, it may be thought, sit well with the mood and views of the House of Lords in *Sidaway*. For she would have the law subordinate the power of the doctor and the autonomy and consent of the child (assuming as we can, I submit, that some children under the age of 16 are perfectly capable of being autonomous) to the authority of the parent.

The argument can be put at least three ways. First a child under the age of 16 is in fact or in law incompetent validly to enter into a relationship as a patient with a doctor. Secondly, a doctor owes no duty to, and cannot treat (save in an emergency) such a child without parental authority, regardless of the child's consent. Thirdly, a parent has a legally recognised right of control over her child until at least the age of 16, which includes control over the child's consulting a doctor. The Secretary of State argued otherwise. A child under the age of 16 can in law, if able to understand what is involved, validly enter into a relationship as a patient. A doctor can, and may indeed be obliged, to treat the child, and a parent's right of control does not extend to forbid the doctor from giving treatment if medically warranted.

For our purposes here the merits of these arguments are not as important as what they represent. There could be no better example of what I have called 'the social process' of determining and delimiting the doctor–patient relationship by recourse to the law than this case. Mrs Gillick has a particular view of family life and the role and rights (as she would assert) of parents. She sees in a doctor's willingness to treat a young girl without parental authority an assault on these parental rights. In other words, medical law, particularly as regards the doctor–patient relationship, both epitomises and represents in microcosm the tension between conflicting social ideologies, just as in *Sidaway* it represented the tension between conflicting views on power in a professional–client relationship. Therefore, the court was pressed by Mrs Gillick to support her view. Whatever view it had taken, the structure and shape of the doctor–patient relationship was being revealed for what it is in essence – an ideological issue.

Data protection

One of the many themes running through the *Gillick* case was that of confidentiality. Was a doctor obliged or entitled to keep secret from parents the fact that a daughter under the age of 16 had consulted him, if she purported to forbid him from telling them? This same issue arose in the *Freeman* case and, indeed, arises in all cases of occupational medicine; namely, the propriety of passing on to the employer information which, *prima facie*, was vouchsafed in confidence.

Here you meet another central strand of the traditional doctor–patient relationship, that, in general terms, third parties are excluded from the relationship, except in rare and well-defined circumstances. The issue of power is again present, this time in the form of the power of the patient to bind the doctor to keep his secrets and the duty and power of the doctor to respect a promise to do so in the face of a desire of a third party, whether an individual or an institution of the State, to know.

Just as Mrs Gillick had argued that a third party (in her case, a parent) had a right to control the creation of a doctor–patient relationship, so, she argued, consistently, information passing between child and doctor should not be, and could not be in law, kept from an interested third party.

The extent to which third parties are entitled to intrude lawfully into the doctor–patient relationship is not, of course, a new problem. The *Gillick* case merely highlights one aspect of what is a continuing debate. In essence there are two issues. The first, which is not for us here, is the question of what happens, or should happen, if the doctor divulges information in circumstances in which it is agreed he was not entitled to. The patient has a remedy in law and the doctor may be cautioned. It is the second issue which we should notice. It concerns the circumstances under which a doctor is obliged to pass on information, despite his (and, obviously, the patient's) unwillingness that he should do so.

This is, self-evidently, again a social and ideological issue concerning the proper bounds of privacy. In the United Kingdom, it is represented as a matter of balance between the principle of respect for privacy and the deemed larger interests of society which may be said to be at stake. I say in the United Kingdom, since in some European countries, notably France and Belgium, the notion of any balance at all is rejected, the view being taken that confidentiality is sacrosanct and admits of no exceptions. Mrs Gillick is claiming that her interest as a parent represents a larger interest which should prevail. The task before the court is to strike the proper balance.

The issue of confidentiality raised in *Gillick* however pales into insignificance when compared with the agonies endured by Parliament in producing the Data Protection Act 1984 to meet the modern realities of electronically stored data. As regards medical information which may be stored electronically, the view was taken very strongly by the medical profession and interested sections of the public, that it should be protected and that others, particularly the police and government departments, should not have access to it, except in very limited and carefully articulated circumstances. Seen from our perspective, this is a statement about the centrality of privacy and confidentiality, and the trust which they engender, to the doctor–patient relationship. What is being said is simply that the doctor–patient relationship as understood at present could not survive if others were allowed access to information given in confidence. And, the argument continues, any revised form of relationship, created under circumstances in which such information was available readily to third parties, would be a worse form, one which would harm the interests of doctor and patient alike.

After much huffing and puffing Parliament conceded this argument. In effect, it conceded, therefore, that the present model of the relationship, at least as regards confidences, is the right one and too valuable an arrangement to tamper with, since more harm than good would flow from it. As a consequence the Department of Health published in mid-1985 a 'Code of Guidance' concerning access to 'health data' which limits disclosure of information largely to those circumstances already recognised by law as justifiable exceptions to the general principle; for example, the reporting of certain diseases or the need to comply with an order of a competent court.

Malpractice

As I have said, medical law is more than malpractice litigation. But, it is of interest to stand back and ask, in what way, if at all, does such litigation bear on what I have suggested is a pressure on the courts to take on the task of defining and reshaping the doctor–patient relationship.

The principal purpose of malpractice litigation is undoubtedly to gain monetary compensation for the party harmed by the negligence of the doctor. But it has another function. This is to serve as a device, the most formal and theoretically the most powerful device, for holding doctors accountable for their conduct. And, of course, accountability, particularly before an external agency, represents a recognition of the potential imbalance of power between the doctor and the patient, and the need to have an institutionalised system to which the patient may have recourse. Other systems exist, of course, ranging from peer review to appearance before the General Medical Council (on which more later). But the lawsuit has, perhaps, the greatest authority.

In every malpractice suit, the court is being asked to call the doctor to account. The very existence of this power in the court, and in the patient to invoke the court's authority, cannot fail to have some important effect on the doctor–patient relationship. It does not, in theory, have to be used a great deal. Indeed, it has not been. That it can be used has traditionally been thought sufficient. It was thought, indeed, that it was better that litigation be relatively uncommon, so that doctors knew that they were subject to the law and the review of the courts, but were not constantly looking over their shoulders for the next lawsuit. Such a state of affairs, many have thought, would deleteriously alter the doctor–patient relationship by making the doctor defensive, by shifting power too much to the patient and thereby frustrating the aim of partnership, as some see happening in the United States.

The difficulty with this appraisal is that it has tended to ignore the fact that malpractice litigation is not, in the event, a very successful way of holding doctors accountable. It depends for its success on patients being able and willing to sue and having evidence which will pass muster and a sympathetic judge. It is no secret that the success rate of litigation against doctors is much lower than in forms of personal injury litigation. This is not to say that the only good system of accountability is one which finds doctors liable. It may, however, encourage doctors to feel that much more secure from the rigours of regulation if they feel that, if sued, they will succeed. And, of course, an often overlooked but critical weakness of this method of accountability is that the cases of egregious conduct which may prompt in the public the legitimate wish to know the doctor involved, if only to avoid him, do not come before the court and public attention. They are settled in private and no one outside a small circle is the wiser.

This realisation that malpractice litigation is not the regulator it could, or should, be, that it is not successfully striking the balance of power between doctor and patient in the way its existence suggests it ought, has produced two developments of interest to us which serve also to confirm the general view I am advancing.

The first is apparently paradoxical. There is a steady but significant increase in litigation. The paradox appears to lie in an increasing resort to a system which is more and more recognised as not producing the desired results. The answer, perhaps, is that the view is hardening in patients and those who advise them that, if it is used more, it will be exposed to greater attention, litigants will develop greater skills, precedents will be built up, and gradually it will be made to work in the way it is supposed to work.

The second development is fascinating. In the face of what I perceive to be growing calls for improvements in the systems for ensuring accountability in doctors, the General Medical Council, which exercises disciplinary powers over the profession, extended in January 1985 the range of its jurisdiction in matters of discipline. The Council redefined that which may amount to 'serious professional misconduct', and thereby come within its jurisdiction. It was decided for the first time that professional incompetence or negligence may amount to serious professional misconduct.

The significance of this development cannot be overstated. A new method of ensuring accountability has been introduced which obviates the need for a lawsuit. The General Medical Council, often, though wrongly, regarded as the medical profession regulating itself (even though it has non-medically qualified members), took the initiative to go beyond consideration of the unethical and the impolite, the alcoholic and adulterous, to adjudicate upon incompetence and thereby hold the scales of power between doctor and patient. Such a development represents some sort of victory for the perception that the doctor–patient relationship is better seen as a partnership, with the patient having proper claims and rights and legitimate expectations, and that a new mechanism to achieve this should be developed. It represents some sort of victory for the proposition that a patient is not to be patronised, or unable to call the doctor to account, by recognising the need for, and establishing, a system to coexist with the courts, designed to set the proper balance of power between doctor and patient. It now remains to be seen how successful it will be.

Conclusion

This social process of defining and reshaping the doctor–patient relationship will continue as attitudes and values change and opinions alter on the proper mechanism for regulation and control. The courts and the law will have a significant role to play, like it or not, and new insights can be gained into legal developments if they are viewed from this perspective.

A SURVEY OF THE YEAR
2. THE LIMITS OF MEDICAL ADVANCE
Peter Byrne

> If a certain medical technology has been developed, it is expected that he the medical practitioner will facilitate his patients' access to it.[1]

This recent remark by a commentator on medical developments records a widely held conviction about the advance of modern medicine. It is to the effect that the greater the advance, the greater will be the human well-being that flows from medicine. There is thus a moral imperative behind the development of medical technique, for the development of technique advances the curative powers of medicine. Hence, human well-being is increased.

Protests against these simple equations have been loudly and eloquently made in medical ethics over the last two decades. What is significant about medical advance during the past year has been the renewed force it has given to such protests and the extent to which it has spread them. In particular, recent controversies surrounding both *in vitro* fertilisation (IVF) and the extension of heart transplant surgery to the very young have shown the strength and extent of the objection to the limitless pursuit of medical advance. The aim of this essay is to indicate by reference to recent literature how these two areas of medicine have raised objections to the moral imperative deemed to be behind the development of medical technique.

Part of the reason why this sort of concern is spreading in this country relates to an issue which continues to be the subject of public debate. The public funding of the National Health Service is producing an increased preoccupation with the comparative costs of what are seen as competing medical techniques. Whether or not government is right in its claim that resources for the NHS are being increased in real terms, the public perception is of a widening gap between available resources and demand throughout the NHS. Given that this gap cannot be bridged in the near future, medical programmes will tend to become competitors whether doctors will or not, and probably judged against each other in terms of such criteria as cost and benefit. If medical advance turns up complex and expensive procedures, they may be judged to be of less value than existing programmes. Thus the paucity of resources can produce circumstances where medical advance becomes morally controversial, if it entails the depletion of funds already stretched and fought over.

The extension of heart transplant surgery

Arguments about medical advance and resources can be taken up immediately in considering public concern over new developments in heart transplant programmes. Among the considerations which limit the doctor's responsibility to apply the techniques of medical science, three can be selected as of particular importance for our discussion. They are: a) the availability of resources, b) the infringement of obligations owed to others, c) the ability to offer a reasonable hope of benefit. The earlier round of heart transplant surgery in the late 1960s and early 1970s gave ground for concern on all three points. There were many who thought that the large sums involved would be better spent elsewhere. Factors a) and b) became linked through the concern that money and manpower were being diverted away from patients for whom less dramatic treatment was possible and desirable. Qualms were felt as to how the acquisition of suitable donor organs was compatible with the obligation of care owed to the donors. The poor survival rate of the recipients of grafted hearts naturally raised the question of whether any reasonable hope of benefit was being offered to the patients. It was asked whether this form of transplant should be regarded more properly as a type of research procedure. This reaction to the early years of heart transplant surgery was a notable instance of the new scepticism about the proper application of medical technology. There was widespread admiration for the skills and techniques involved, and equally widespread doubt whether they were worth pursuing.

The subsequent programme of transplant surgery that began in the late 1970s at Papworth and Harefield hospitals has aroused similar but more muted protests. The financial needs of the transplant programme were adversely commented on by a consultant cardiologist, Dr D W Evans:

> ... the Papworth programme is estimated to have cost £644,735 so far, whereas the donated money amounts to £400,000. Approval for the programme was understood to be conditional upon its making no extra charge upon the strained local health budget.[2]

Dr Evans also objected to the taking of organs from donors whom he regarded as still alive. This objection is now shared by few owing to the widespread acceptance of brain-stem death as an adequate definition of death. Overall, such doubts about the renewed programme have not been influential, simply because of the success of the latest surgery in giving a real expectation of benefit. With the development in Cambridge of a more effective drug (cyclosporin) to combat tissue rejection, it is estimated that the chances of surviving for twelve months after the graft of a new heart are better than 8 in 10, and for those who pass that hurdle the five-year survival rate is expected to be 90 per cent.

In August and October 1984 heart transplant programmes in this country and America respectively took a dramatic new turn with the extension of the operation to the new-born. First Hollie Roffey was given a new heart by the surgeon in charge of the Harefield unit, Mr Magdi Yacoub. Then at the Loma Linda Medical Center in California, Dr Leonard Bailey performed a heart transplant operation on a new-born who has come to be known as Baby Fae. Neither child survived for more than a few days. The operation on Baby Fae attracted most comment because of the bizarre circumstances surrounding it. Dr Bailey chose to transplant a baboon's heart into the infant. It was alleged by some that he did not seek a suitable human organ, nor proper informed consent from the parents. In all the circumstances his statement that this was not experiment for experiment's sake is unlikely to have persuaded many.[3]

The theatricality surrounding the case of Baby Fae is incidental to the main issues arising from the extension of major transplant surgery to the very young. Once again the British case raised the question of the proper use of limited financial resources. Professor Michael Oliver, president of the British Cardiac Society, said: 'The procedure and the maintenance of a normal life after the replacement of an infant's heart are such formidable calls upon resources that their place in the responsible delivery of health care must be questioned'.[4] But whilst this is no doubt an important consideration, those who followed the last days of Hollie Roffey and Baby Fae will be more concerned with the *human* costs of the surgery in relation to expected benefit. Amongst the human costs must be reckoned the distress and discomfort of the operation itself, the harmful effects of the immuno-suppressive drugs, and the pain and discomfort of taking blood samples and performing other tests. And there is the anguish and distress of the parents whose hopes are first raised and then dashed. A leading transplant surgeon commented:

> All these factors must be taken into account, and while an adult may be able to appreciate and accept them, a child cannot easily do so, and the quality of life for a child with an organ graft can be very unsatisfactory. The writer is therefore reluctant to perform organ grafting in young children although parents frequently request it as a last resort.[5]

The logical outcome of this line of reasoning on the human costs of heart transplant surgery on infants is the acceptance of the death of the infants. Professor Oliver, noting that 'embryological development is not always perfect', points the moral very clearly:

> Surgeons, physicans and parents should learn to accept that biology can go awry and that technical feats may not right it again. In the context of malformed hearts incompatible with prolonged survival, many parents are young enough to try again.[6]

In operating upon Hollie Roffey, Mr Yacoub was obviously confident that technical feats would one day be able to right biology. By way of defending his decision, he pointed to two factors which had made such operations feasible. The first was the development of new immuno-suppressive drugs which enabled the baby's rejection response to be overcome without the use of harmful steroids that might otherwise hinder normal growth. The second factor was evidence from research into transplants on young animals, and the transplant of children's hearts into adults, indicating that the three-day-old heart placed in Hollie could, in principle, be expected to grow and develop. However, it is evident that, despite these advances, the operation upon Hollie was very much an experimental procedure. Mr Yacoub said:

> We have done a lot of work and preparation and everything suggested to us that it should work. Now Hollie has answered some of the unknowns for us.[7]

The parents were told, said Mr Yacoub, 'that they were going into the unknown. The parents were very keen and Hollie's mother said that if Hollie did not make it she would at least benefit others'. So we have a medical procedure which is feasible in principle, but which was applied to a new-born baby with only a slim chance of her gaining any lasting benefit. However, she definitely made a contribution to the advance of knowledge, albeit unknowingly.

Some would say that any chance of life is better than no chance at all. They would conclude that Baby Fae and Hollie Roffey were offered real benefits. Yet it is hard to accept either the premise or conclusion of this argument. The cost of the slim chance of life matters. The chance of life is not a good that will outweigh all the evils that may be involved in buying it. The two babies seemed to have been the subjects of procedures whose main justification lay in the knowledge they could contribute to later transplant attempts, thus providing a further objection to this extension of the heart transplant programme. If we accept the principle that children may not be 'volunteered' for experimental procedures, otherwise unjustifiable for the benefit they bring to their subjects, then we have ground for saying that, though the technology of heart transplants for the very young exists, it ought to be kept on the shelf for the time being. The ethical principle appealed to here derives from the more fundamental claim that, where the point of a medical procedure is largely experimental, it cannot be undertaken without the explicit and informed consent of the patient. Presumed or proxy consent will not do, because they are only appropriate for treatments which any normal or reasonable person would assent to in the circumstances. It cannot be assumed that any normal or reasonable person would assent to pioneer surgery offering the balance between benefit and harm we see here.

It may be objected that the first babies who receive heart transplants are by definition pioneers. All first operations are experimental procedures. If pioneering work is ruled out as unethical, the cure will *always* remain on the shelf. The reply must be that while logically there have to be some pioneers if techniques are ever to become established, this must not entail pioneers entering the lists with the odds stacked so heavily against them. We should expect to see much more collateral work done on heart transplants before young babies are selected for surgery. It is not for a layman to specify the further research needed. No doubt it will include more information from the treatment of older patients and from animal experiments (presuming the latter to be licit). We hope for a time where heart transplants for babies will be not merely feasible (Mr Yacoub's word) but will offer a substantial expectation of benefit. Many will feel that they should not recommence until collateral work enables surgeons to offer substantial benefits.

Artificial aids to reproduction

The various ethical, legal and medical issues surrounding the development of artificial aids to reproduction have been the subject of public discussion for some time, but during the past year they have come to a head with a number of key developments. These include: the publication of the Warnock report (*Report of the Committee of Inquiry into Human Fertilisation and Embryology*, Cmnd. 9314), the debate on Mr Enoch Powell's 'Unborn Children (Protection) Bill', the first surrogate birth in this country and the appearance of a wide range of books and studies on the ethics of assisted reproduction.

The moral doubts over the techniques involved are, in sum, that they have led to an improper interference in the creation of life and will further lead to a morally objectionable manipulation of human life. In general, these techniques have led medicine into a sphere which is not its proper concern and where it can gain no sanction from the accepted moral imperatives to treat and cure. The importance of the debate over the techniques of assisted reproduction is reflected in the space devoted to it in later chapters of this volume. I shall accordingly limit my discussion to the issues surrounding *in vitro* fertilisation (IVF). My aim is to categorise and survey the most important objections offered against it with a view to seeing if a case has been made for supposing that medical advance in this instance passes beyond the bounds of moral acceptability.

Within the great mass of comment on IVF and assisted reproduction there are four main types of moral objection to the procedures involved.

1. Artificially induced fertilisation is wrong in itself.
2. Treatment of infertility by such means is not a proper medical goal.
3. Research on embryos involved in IVF or arising out of it is wrong in itself.
4. Research on embryos is being, or will be, used for improper purposes.

This list of objections is not meant to cover all those to be found in the literature, but I consider them to be the most important. A discussion of such a bald summary of qualms about IVF and assisted reproduction cannot begin to provide an exhaustive or complete answer to all the social and ethical issues raised, but it can indicate the importance of the debate for the conduct of medical advance.

It reveals the marked ambiguity in public attitudes to medical research and its application. For some, the doctor may not be seen as healer but as an improper manipulator of human life and its origins. The debate is also noteworthy for what it reveals about the disagreements within our society, and our inability to resolve those disagreements in a way which may be perceived as authoritative. This difficulty reflects upon the limits of medical advance, for it points to the problem of providing medical science with a sure moral context in which to conduct its research. It is noticeable in this regard that the Warnock report, though commissioned by government, was not seen as a resolution of the issues surrounding IVF and related techniques. It became, rather, just another controversial contribution to a continuing debate. Mr Powell's Bill was in fact founded upon a rejection of some of the report's main recommendations (those in chapter 11 on the licitness of research on embryos up to 14 days old). The Warnock report itself contained significant minority dissent on the question of embryo research (and on surrogacy).

I now turn to a consideration of the four main objections I have listed above.

1. 'Artificially induced fertilisation is wrong in itself'. This objection may be made against various forms of assisted reproduction, but it is particularly aroused by IVF because it is a technique involving fertilisation outside the female body and through the manipulation of ovum and sperm by the doctor or scientist. Thus the way is open to making an easy contrast between the natural begetting of children and their manufacture by medicine. The contrast is usually made so as to condemn IVF. 'Is there not a danger that human procreation is being reduced to battery farming?' ask critics of 'the concept that we can "manufacture" human beings.'[8] This contrast between natural begetting and artificial manufacture is at the heart of Oliver O'Donovan's critique of IVF in *Begotten or Made?*[1] How cogent an objection to artificially assisted pregnancy lies behind the contrast is a matter for debate. I would note, however, one substantive point that could lie behind the, at least in part, rhetorical opposition between begetting and manufacturing. Objection to IVF and other techniques may be made on the ground that artificially induced conception disrupts intercourse–conception–pregnancy and thus destroys the unity of the act of procreation and love within marriage, a point clearly made in the Catholic bishops' submission to the Warnock committee.[9] The following argument from John Mahoney may be sufficient answer:

> It is clear that the production of a child should be expressive of the loving interchange between husband and wife, and not just an impersonal, clinical contribution by each of the ingredients required for conception ... But it is equally clear that the frustrations of childless couples and all the disruption

and inconvenience entailed by clinical procedures for ... *in vitro* fertilisation can also be expressions of deep mutual love and of a shared longing to give each other a child as a fruit of their married life.[10]

An IVF child can still be the expression of marital loving actions, even though the expression cannot exist without the help of medical science.

John Mahoney concludes that procedures such as IVF are in themselves neither moral nor immoral. They acquire a moral character only within a context. Society needs a view on who may properly be given artificial help in procreation and for what reasons. (There is some comment on these two vital issues in the Warnock report, pages 10–12.) If the application of IVF is regulated by firm answers to these questions, it may be concluded that, for all the complaints about 'manufacturing' children, IVF need not flout such positive views about the nature of procreation, marriage and child-rearing as society still possesses.

2. 'Treatment of infertility by such means is not a proper medical goal'. My statement of this objection endeavours to catch the spirit of a point against assisted reproduction that can be found in one contribution to the Council for Science and Society's *Human Procreation: Ethical Aspects of the New Techniques*[11] and in *Begotten or Made?*[12] The argument is that IVF is neither a treatment nor a cure for infertility. It is a means of compensation for infertility or circumventing it through artificial help in commencing a pregnancy. But to be childless is not to be ill, and if medical science provides women with pregnancies it does not fulfil a medical goal; it provides a social service in meeting the socially acquired need of a couple to have a child and, in doing so, forfeits the sanction which lies behind normal acts of treatment or cure. In these circumstances, the moral imperative behind applying and funding medical advance fails.

Those who advance this kind of argument strike me as having failed to see the close parallel that can exist between IVF treatment and other forms of medical compensation for the results of bodily damage or disease. They also ignore the variety of reasons there might be behind claims for assisted procreation. Someone who has lost a limb is not ill and medicine can offer no treatment or cure. But he is hindered in the full enjoyment of life or the full exercise of normal human capacities. The provision of an artificial limb is not 'treatment' which makes him 'well', the damage is not removed, but he is provided with a means of circumventing the harmful effects of his loss. Can anyone doubt that this is medically worthwhile, to be supported by society at large? It is difficult to see why the provision of IVF to a couple whose female partner has diseased or damaged fallopian tubes should be viewed differently. Such infertility is the result of bodily damage or disease. If medical science can compensate for it, the support of society in developing and applying the means of compensation should be forthcoming.

There are better grounds for this argument when considering the use of IVF and other techniques to provide a child for a lesbian couple. No matter how desirable such a service might be, there is some point in saying that it is not a medical service, nor offered in pursuit of a medical goal. It cannot claim the sanction that lies behind the treatment, or cure or compensation for bodily damage. There is a need to consider the context before judging the moral character of IVF and other forms of artificial aids to procreation.

3. 'Research on embryos involved in or arising out of IVF is wrong in itself'. The development of IVF techniques in this country, in Australia and elsewhere has involved research upon early embryos. The practice of IVF frequently entails the creation of 'spare' embryos (that is, embryos which will not be re-implanted) to increase the chances of successful fertilisation *in vitro*. These 'spare' embryos will then be available for a variety of research purposes. Embryos may indeed be deliberately created from donated ova for the purposes of research. Regarding the early embryo as having a moral claim which forbids experiment upon it is a decisive reason for rejecting IVF.

How far this argument *does* provide a decisive objection to IVF is not clear. A number of questions need to be considered. Could research for perfecting the techniques of IVF as a treatment for infertility be done satisfactorily on animal embryos? Would it be proper to extract on each occasion fewer ova from women undergoing IVF treatment in order to avoid the creation of 'spare' embryos, although at the cost of further episodes of treatment? I must leave such questions open but note that those involved in the development of IVF techniques are of the opinion that some research on human embryos is required and that it would be improper in the light of obligations owed to patients to limit the extraction of ova so as to rule out 'spares'. These matters remain contested.

If it is assumed, for the sake of argument, that IVF does involve some form of experimental work on human embryos, what is to be made of the objection that such research is illicit and IVF in consequence morally questionable? Here we must distinguish between differing views of the moral status of the embryo. One view is implied in the title of Mr Powell's bill: from the moment of fertilisation the embryo is an unborn child, to be protected from procedures not designed to benefit it, exactly as a human infant is protected. The majority view of the Warnock committee is that before the significant differentiation of embryonic tissue, which they place at 14 days, the embryo although it enjoys special status, is not to be considered a human person. If research is subject to 'stringent controls and monitoring' and is in the interests of advancing medical knowledge and treatment, it may override the claim of the embryo upon us.[14] Two minority reports from the Warnock committee offer shades of opinion between the view that the embryo is at all times an unborn child and the view of the majority. One argues that the special status of the embryo forbids the deliberate manufacture of embryos for research[15]; the other contends that the early embryo has at all times the *potential* for humanness and for this reason can never licitly be a subject for research.[16]

In describing these four opinions about the status of the embryo and the licitness of using it for research I have only hinted at the complexities of opinion expressed on these matters. No attempt can be offered in these pages to decide the question of the moral status of the embryo. I would suggest, however, that we need to reflect not so much on this question directly but more on the matter of which view of the status of the embryo should be normative for *society*, granted that even though *personal* opinions may differ some overall consensus could be achieved. It is the view of society that will be vital in deciding upon the funding or licensing of future research. If society can reach a consensus on these matters, it will not be through the elimination of strongly held personal views on the status of embryonic life, but through the discovery of a set of opinions which a majority of those concerned are prepared to accept as a working compromise. This may then become the basis of social policy. Resources for constructing such a compromise can be found in existing practices towards embryonic life and in the historical roots of our ethical thought. Significant elements in present practice and in the history of Western thought on the status of the embryo seem to me to point away from the view that embryos are 'unborn children'.

On the score of practice I would point to the wide acceptance of inter-uterine contraceptive devices as means of family planning. Objections cannot disguise the social consensus that they are acceptable, yet their use involves the destruction of embryonic life. They prevent implantation of the embryo; they do not prevent contraception. In Western thought, the view that the human embryo enjoys the moral status of a human infant from its earliest moments is a recent phenomenon, as is evident from the Chief Rabbi's contribution to this volume, from Gordon Dunstan's essay in the Council for Science and Society's report[17] and from John Mahoney's *Bioethics and Belief*.[18] It remained a minority view even amongst the Christian churches until the nineteenth century. If we are true to our moral past, which of course we need not be, we may give the embryo a special status but not the status of a human infant.

Historical reflection having led us this far, we might conclude that although the early embryo has a dignity, a worth, it is not fully equivalent to the dignity of a person and, therefore, that research on embryos is in principle licit up to a certain point of development. Society could rightly view the claims of the embryo and the claims of research as incompatible and, theoretically, accept that the dignity of the embryo should give way to other claims. Society would not rule out research but would be alert to its purposes and the kinds of human needs and values behind it. It would weigh the dignity of the embryo against the worth of such needs and values. It would not ban research but regulate it. These remarks leave untouched the question of whether embryos could ever licitly be specially created for the purposes of research.

4. 'Reseach on embryos is being, or will be, used for improper purposes'. Those who practice research on embryos appear to justify their purposes by referring to the authority enjoyed by other forms of research seeking to treat or compensate for disease or disability. They say their purposes include: improving treatment and compensation for infertility; diagnosing and preventing chromasomal abnormalities resulting in spontaneous abortions, in Down's syndrome or in Turner's syndrome; aiding the very early diagnosis of genetically related disorders. Critics of IVF cite other purposes, however. For example, the Order of Christian Unity, at its London conference in May 1984, informed the world of such likely purposes as sex selection, breeding human beings to specification, and growing human embryos in other species. It also asked: if embryos could be bred outside the womb for up to 14 days or more, why scientists should not want to breed for up to 60 days and eventually to term?[19]

With these abuses in mind it is to be expected that embryo research will be associated with the activities of concentration camp doctors in the Third Reich (as was done at the OCU conference). It is doubtful how far the listing of actual or possible abuses should determine a view of the licitness of embryo research and the techniques which make it possible. To condemn something because it *could* be abused, to conclude that what *could* happen *will* happen, may seem a very odd way of proceeding. It can be argued that to condemn IVF and its associated procedures on account of these possible abuses is in fact to condemn ourselves: for it is to predict that we will be unable to give these medical advances an appropriate legal and ethical context.

Reflecting on the limits of medical advance provided by the examples considered in this essay points to an important moral. The limits of proper advance in medicine can never be set simply by what is technically possible. They must also be set by a legal and ethical context which will consider the social and human benefits of medical advance in relation to its costs and be attentive to the purposes behind medical advance. The creation of such a context will ensure that medical advance is indeed human advance.

Notes and references

1 O O'Donovan. Begotten or made? Oxford, Oxford University Press, 1984, page 9.
2 Letter, The Times, 13 September 1982.
3 The Times, 17 November 1984.
4 The Times, 30 November 1984.
5 R Y Calne. Tissue transplant. In: A S Duncan, G R Dunstan and T R Wellbourne (eds). A dictionary of medical ethics. London, Darton Longman and Todd, 1981, page 437.
6 The Times, 30 November 1984.
7 Interview, The Sunday Times, 19 August 1984. The comments that follow are all taken from this interview.
8 Sir Bernard Braine and Lord Robertson of Oakridge. Letter, The Times, 6 June 1984.
9 See In vitro fertilisation: morality and public policy. Catholic Information Services, 1983, sections 20ff.
10 John Mahoney. Bioethics and belief: religion and medicine in dialogue. London, Sheed and Ward, 1984, page 17.
11 Council for Science and Society. Human procreation: ethical aspects of the new techniques. Oxford, Oxford University Press, 1984, page 60.
12 See 1 above, pages 28ff.
13 See the statement of R G Edwards and P C Steptoe, letter, The Times, 6 June 1984.
14 Department of Health and Social Security. Report of the Committee of Inquiry into Human Fertilisation and Embryology. Cmnd 9314 (Chairman: Dame Mary Warnock) London, HMSO, 1984, page 64.
15 See 14 above, page 94.

16 See 14 above, pages 90–93.
17 See 11 above, Introduction pages 1–11.
18 See 10 above, pages 57–59.
19 As reported in The Times and The Guardian, 22 May 1984.

RE-READING WARNOCK

Simon Lee

At its worst, the Warnock report[1] was the product of the wrong people considering the wrong issues in the wrong way. At its best it provides pointers to good medical law, ethics and practice. In order to separate the good from the bad and indeed from the downright ugly, this article suggests re-reading the report in a particular order, looking out for unanswered and even unasked questions.

1. Team and tactics

The first pages to read are those listing the members of the committee.[2] The team you pick and the task you give them obviously determine the result. As a nine-year-old, I could have told Alf Ramsey that he should have selected Jimmy Greaves for the England World Cup Final side in 1966 and that he should have employed more attacking tactics. Ever since, I have preferred my imaginary selections and tactics to those actually chosen for England soccer, rugby and cricket teams. Before selecting my ideal Warnock committee I must admit that, my views notwithstanding, Alf Ramsey's side did win the World Cup. But the importance of the role which faced Warnock makes it worthwhile to question the membership of the committee even if our own preferences can be dismissed as subjective or misguided.

How many of the sixteen members can you name? Why were they on the committee? Why were more illustrious experts not on the committee? The nucleus of my preferred composition can be found elsewhere in the pages of the report, in the list of those submitting evidence.[3] I would have included doctors and scientists working within the field of *in vitro* fertilisation such as Edwards, Steptoe, Craft and Winston. Then I would have chosen lawyers and philosophers with a special interest in medical law and ethics such as Kennedy, Finnis, Hoggett, Dunstan, Mahoney and Glover. Most of those either gave evidence in their own right or by helping to draft the submissions of organisations. But in order to use their expertise within the committee, we also have to reconsider the role allotted to the inquiry.

Those who have devoted considerable professional attention to the topic in hand are unlikely to be picked for an offical committee because their views are known in advance and known to conflict. Yet this is only a problem if the committee is expected to produce unanimous or majority recommendations, whereas a far more useful role for such committees is to pave the way for public and parliamentary debate by presenting, in a detailed, comprehensible way, the best arguments for and against the plausible alternative courses of action. The individual members' preferences do not need to be recorded. It is for the rest of society to decide which way to proceed on the basis of the experts' analysis of the issues.

Now the Warnock committee itself is not to blame for its different approach since its terms of reference directed it to make recommendations. No doubt this helps the government pass the buck of responsibility for controversial proposals, but it diverts the inquiry's energy away from the arguments and towards the vagueness which can command wider assent. Moreover, it makes the government wary of appointing experts. My own selection would be rounded off with an eminent surgeon specialising in a different area; a GP, a psychologist and a social worker, all with experience of counselling infertile couples; someone representing infertile couples themselves and someone who had participated in *in vitro* fertilisation as a donor. Some of these were on the Warnock committee but it is the absence of people like Edwards and Kennedy which is to be regretted. Equally regrettable is the emphasis on what any group of sixteen would themselves prefer, instead of using their expertise to enlighten and involve all of us.

2. Evidence

Our second port of call is the Appendix to the report – perhaps the most interesting part – which lists organisations and individual experts who gave evidence to the committee. Apart from civil service briefing and the committee's own research, this is the key to the information on which the inquiry came to its conclusions. The appendix is a fascinating list of concerned bodies. Some idea of the variety of viewpoints can be gleaned from an alphabetical selection of eye-catching titles: Action for Lesbian Parents; British Toxicology Society; Campaign for Homosexual Equality – Tyneside Group; Donors' Offspring; Episcopal Church in Scotland; Free Church of Scotland; Guild of Catholic Doctors; High Court of Justice – Family Division; Institute of Marital Studies; Justices' Clerks' Society; Knights of St Columbanus – Northern Area Committee; League of Jewish Women; Mothers' Union; National Association of Ovulation Method Instructors; Presbyterian Church of Ireland; Responsible Society; Science Fiction Foundation; Trades Union Congress; United Kingdom Islamic Mission; Voluntary Council for Handicapped Children; West Indian Standing Conference; and the Yorkshire Pro-Life Co-ordinating Committee. Even this wide range of organisations did not satisfy the committee which recorded 'with regret that we did not receive evidence from as wide a range of minority and special interest groups as we would have liked, despite our best endeavours'.

Twenty organisations or individuals were asked to give oral evidence, presumably because the committee was particularly impressed by their written submissions or by their reputation. Clearly the committee considered Northern Ireland in depth since among the fourteen oral submissions from organisations more than half were from Ulster: Association of District Committees for the Health and Personal Social Services, Northern Ireland, Health and Social Services Boards (Northern Ireland), Eastern Incorporated Law Society of Northern Ireland, Methodist Church in Ireland, National Association for the Childless (Northern Ireland), Northern Ireland Council for Nurses and Midwives, Presbyterian Church of Ireland, Ulster Obstetrical and Gynaecological Society.

It would have been interesting to learn which evidence the committee found persuasive and indeed what the evidence was.

This would, of course, have been a gigantic exercise but it is intriguing to wonder if anybody supported some of the more outlandish possible future developments to which we shall shortly turn. In any event, the appendix is undoubtedly worth reading after examining the list of members.

3. Infertility

Where next after the beginning and the end of the report? Well, the terms of reference are set out in paragraph 1.2. as follows:

> To consider recent and potential developments in medicine and science related to human fertilisation and embryology; to consider what policies and safeguards should be applied, including consideration of the social, ethical and legal implications of these developments; and to make recommendations.

The report, however, seems to take as its focus infertility. Chapter 2 is headed 'Infertility: The Scope and Organisation of Services' and the next six chapters concern 'Techniques for the Alleviation of Infertility'. We are not offered a definition of infertility, nor are its causes explained, nor are treatments other than *in vitro* fertilisation discussed. If the inquiry was to focus on infertility, these should surely have been three initial matters of vital significance. The Catholic Bishops' Joint Committee on Bio-Ethical Issues, in contrast, has noted:[4]

> ... the Report's striking silence about the causes of infertility, and its consequent failure to consider how social policy might seek to reduce infertility by attending to its causes. *In vitro* fertilisation (IVF), when used as a clinical technique, is largely designed to solve those problems of infertility which are caused by tubal occlusion. But the commonest causes of tubal occlusion (accounting for about 90% of cases) are previous abortion, the use of the IUD as a contraceptive device, and sexually transmitted diseases. To have pointed to these causes would have taken courage. It would not, however, have implied that all cases of infertility result from such avoidable causes. And what is at stake is a matter of fact, of truths which it is irresponsible for society to conceal from its vulnerable members. Public policy should

not ignore these facts when determining the proper distribution of society's inevitably limited resources for health-care.

'Are the bishops right?' and 'If so, so what?' are important questions which merit answers but which Warnock fails even to ask. Society certainly should ask whether prevention is better than cure (or, rather 'alleviation').

4. Eligibility

The report *does* ask who should be eligible for infertility treatment but we are not really given the reasons for the committee's conclusions, which are: '... we believe that as a general rule it is better for children to be born into a two-parent family, with both father and mother'[5] but '... we are not prepared to recommend that access to treatment should be based exclusively on the legal status of marriage.'[6] So the question for us is whether only 'good' prospective parents should be eligible. If so, does 'good' mean married, or at least a couple, or at the very least heterosexual? The report is tantalising in raising questions about the eligibility of single homosexuals but ultimately failing to counter the argument that 'a single person, whether man or woman, can in certain circumstances provide a suitable environment for a child, since the existence of single adoptive parents is specifically provided for in the Children Act 1975.'[7] Clearly, artificial insemination by a donor and surrogate motherhood provide opportunities for the single heterosexual person and, perhaps more intriguingly, the lesbian or homosexual couple to 'start a family' in a way which may challenge traditional notions of the family.

Within heterosexual relationships, the report's rejection of marriage as the dividing-line for eligibility will annoy some and please others. But both groups might have expected more discussion of the arguments about whether a child's best interests are served by being born of or for a married couple. A serious question which the report raises but again fails to resolve adequately is whether a couple with a previous conviction for child abuse should be ineligible for infertility treatment. A final point in this context is the question of priorities in a world of scarce resources. Should treatment be available to those who earlier opted for infertility through sterilisation but (perhaps after remarrying) have now changed their minds, or to those who have become involuntarily infertile but who already have children?

5. Donors

In this idiosyncratic meander through the Warnock report, I next suggest turning to paragraph 4.21. Apart from being intrinsically interesting, its recommendation has the distinction of being omitted from the original copies of the report. It now appears as Recommendation 20[8] and the subsequent proposals are accordingly renumbered. This has caused minimal confusion though doubtless maximum concern to the HMSO proof-readers.

> 4.21. As a matter of principle we do not wish to encourage the possibility of prospective parents seeking donors with specific characteristics by the use of whose semen they hope to give birth to a particular type of child. We do not therefore want detailed descriptions of donors to be used as a basis for choice, but we believe that the couple should be given sufficient relevant information for their reassurance. This should include some basic factors about the donor, such as his ethnic group and his genetic health. A small minority of the Inquiry, while supporting the principle set out above, and without compromising the principle of anonymity, consider that a gradual move towards making more detailed descriptions of the donor available to prospective parents, if requested, could be beneficial to the practice of AID, provided this was accompanied by appropriate counselling. We recommend that on reaching the age of eighteen the child should have access to the basic information about the donor's ethnic origin and genetic health and that legislation be enacted to provide the right of access to this. This legislation should not be retrospective.

What is the principle which matters at the beginning of this quotation and why doesn't the committee argue the pros and cons of any such principle? Is it wrong for spouses to choose each other partly with a view to their genetic contribution to children of the marriage? Is that an anologous issue? If the donor's 'ethnic group' is a 'basic fact' then why not his height, hair or eye colour, intelligence and so on? Is the report pandering to racial prejudice or is it just being sensible? A final point of interest in the paragraph is the reference to a 'small minority of the Inquiry'. How small and, given the attention to majorities and minorities elsewhere in the report, why are we not told the numbers? As I have already indicated, I am personally unmoved by the numbers debate so I would prefer to hear the *arguments* which this small minority and its opposing large majority have to offer.

6. *Experimenting on embryos*

Lest it be thought that I have at last reached what is taken to be the central question of the embryo's status, I am here rather drawing attention to the question: what is meant by *experimenting* on embryos? For some, any research on embryos is unacceptable since it uses them as a means to an end. Others, however, may suspend judgement until they have an idea of what it means to experiment on embryos. Paragraph 11.10 begins by raising the hope that it will explain 'experiment' but then discusses a different aspect. So at no point in the report is there an explanation of what embryo experiments entail.

Taking the analogy of the comatose adult patient, while no one would countenance evil doctors dismembering 'to see what happens', many would have no objection to doctors sitting at the bedside and simply watching to see if they can gain any insights for the future. If embryo experiments involve sticking sharp instruments into the embryo, more opposition will form than if they involve observing development through a microscope. As it happens, I would still object, but I suspect an explanation of what constitutes research on embryos would have won more converts to the Warnock majority acceptance of some experiment.

My preferred outcome would be a ban on the creation of so-called 'spare' embryos, or of embryos destined only for experiment, so that the problem of how to treat them does not arise; but a related point of importance for the Warnock majority is what happens to the embryo when the experiments have to stop after 14 days. Again, the report does not explain their fate but one imagines that they are flushed down a sink or incinerated. Is this any more respectful of their 'special status' than another day of experiment?

7. Morality and law

The final preliminary issues which the Warnock report should have clarified were its attitude to theories of morality and its approach to the relationship between law and morality. On morality, the key recommendation of paragraph 11.18 with its utilitarian approach should be contrasted with the damning indictment of utilitarianism contained in paragraph 4 of the Foreword and in paragraph 8.17.

> [Pro-utilitarian] 11.18. We do not want to see a situation in which human embryos are frivolously or unnecessarily used in research but we are bound to take account of the fact that the advances in the treatment of infertility, which we have discussed in the earlier part of this report, could not have taken place without such research; and that continued research is essential, if advances in treatment and medical knowledge are to continue. A majority of us therefore agreed that research on human embryos should continue.

> [Anti-utilitarian] Paragraph 4, Foreword A strict utilitarian would suppose that, given certain procedures, it would be possible to calculate their benefits and their costs. Future advantages, therapeutic or scientific, should be weighed against present and future harm. However, even if such a calculation were possible, it could not provide a final or verifiable answer to the question whether it is right that such procedures should be carried out. There would still remain the possibility that they were unacceptable, whatever their long-term benefits were supposed to be. Moral questions, such as those with which we have been concerned are, by definition, questions that involve not only a calculation of consequences, but also strong sentiments with regard to the nature of the proposed activities themselves.

[Anti-utilitarian] 8.17. That people should treat others as a means to their own ends, however desirable the consequences, must always be liable to moral objection.

As far as the relationship between morality and law is concerned, the report must again be dubbed inconsistent. Paragraph 4.16 on artificial insemination by a donor should be contrasted with paragraphs 8.17 and 8.18 on surrogate motherhood. Those who object to sperm (and, elsewhere, egg or embryo) donation are told that they should not impose their moral standpoint on those who disagree, but a majority of the committee is prepared to ban surrogate agencies when the same point could be made. The report does not explain how to bridge the gap from deciding that something is immoral to deciding that it should be illegal.

8. *Hamstermen*

When re-reading Warnock, therefore, I would focus on the questions of membership, methodology, evidence, infertility, eligibility, donors, experiment, morality and law before turning to the 'recent and potential developments' which the committee's terms of reference concerned. I would then begin with the potential rather than the recent, concentrating on paragraphs 12.2, 3, 5 and 9. We already have embryo experiments and surrogate motherhood but there is a chance that we can stop unacceptable future developments if we act now. Moreover, what seems implausible today may well be achieved, if not tomorrow, at least within a decade, for in this area 'medical science ... may advance with startling rapidity' (paragraph 1.9).

So the first substantive question to face under this scheme is whether to allow the development of Hamstermen[9] or, more probably, Gorillamen. Hitherto unshockably liberal students have unanimously drawn the line at this point in my experience of discussing the Warnock report. I have yet to meet any person (or indeed any hamster or gorilla) who has expressed acceptance of such developments beyond the two-cell stage. But why do we object to trans-species fertilisation involving humans? Are farming techniques which cross-fertilise non-human species also unacceptable? Are we speciesists and, if so, is there anything wrong in such an attitude?

We seem to share an intuition to protect the boundaries of our species or, as it is often expressed, to preserve the Dignity of Humanity. As Ian Kennedy might say, this is the 'yuck' factor. Our response is one of disgust and that itself is significant. If forced to rationalise this emotional reaction, we may flounder but that does not necessarily invalidate the intuition.

Paragraph 12.9 moves on to ban the placing of a human embryo in the uterus of another species for gestation. While the report thinks of this practice as only a 'possibility', other evidence suggests that it is already happening. Who wants camels as surrogate mothers? Again, I suspect many regard Warnock's recommendation as correctly reflecting a general repugnance at such an idea. On the other hand, Warnock does not *argue* for this view. Is the statement of moral intuition enough? On both trans-species fertiliation and gestation, I suspect most people regard argument as unnecessary. That may be because the argument is obvious, although not to everyone, but it may be because we have reached the limits of rationality's usefulness.

The third issue in Chapter 12 to which I wish to draw attention is 'the use of human embryos for testing drugs etc.' Paragraph 12.5. reads as follows, emphasis added:

> Use of human embryos for testing drugs etc.
> 12.5 It has been suggested that human embryos could be used to test the effects of new developed drugs or other substances that may possibly be toxic or cause abnormalities. This is an area that causes deep concern because of the possibility of mass production of *in vitro* embryos, perhaps on a commercial basis for these purposes. We feel very strongly that the routine testing of drugs on human embryos is not an acceptable area of research *because this would require the manufacture of large numbers of embryos. We concluded however that there may be very particular cirucmstances where the testing of such substances on a very small scale may be justifiable.*

The ridiculousness of this numbers game has been well chronicled.[10] For our purposes, let us accept Warnock's very strong feeling against the routine testing of drugs on human embryos and ask whether this means that feelings are sufficient warrant for action in themselves and whether the real reason behind such feelings is inconsistent with allowing *any* experiments on embryos.

9. Embryo experiments[11] and surrogate motherhood[12]

Having re-read, or perhaps read for the first time, various hitherto obscure parts of the report, it is finally time to turn to the issues which have dominated media reaction to Warnock. It is for each of us to reflect on these questions and come to our own conclusions. One or two pointers have emerged which may bear repetition. Certainly, there is no need to feel that the conclusion of the Warnock majority (9–7) on embryo experiments[13] has any special authority. With different members, the majority could easily have swung the other way and in any case we should be more interested in the arguments underpinning the competing views. Nor is there any need to feel that the majority's utilitarianism should prevail over a rights-based approach to morality. Nor should we underestimate the importance of our feelings, whether they concern Hamstermen, surrogate motherhood or embryo experiments.

While I hope to have nudged the reader in the 'right' critical direction, it is not my intention here to rehearse my own views on embryo experiments and surrogate motherhood.[14] Instead, I have aimed to regenerate interest in reading and reflecting on the whole of the Warnock report. Rather than constantly re-reading the conclusions on one or two issues, there is more to gain by a fresh approach to the questions outlined above. To end on a note of praise for Warnock, however, we should turn to yet another neglected part of the report - the final chapter which recommends a quango to oversee *in vitro* fertilisation.

10. Warnock's legacy to medical law and ethics

Medical law and ethics is all the rage. Warnock, Gillick, Sage (kidney dialysis) and Sidaway (informed consent) have all hit the 1985 headlines. Unfortunately we have no one suitable forum for structuring debate, educating a fascinated public and providing authoritative guidance on these vital issues.

The courts, for instance, can only provide sporadic *ex post factors* review of problems, depending on the vagaries of litigation, nor is the traditional English court procedure appropriate to consider the vast amount of scientific, medical, moral and economic evidence which is germane to, say, the question of allocating kidney dialysis machines. The long-running Gillick saga illustrates another disadvantage of course: as appeal follows appeal there is often confusion and uncertainty.

The Warnock committee could have been a more encouraging model but, apart from the faults noted above, it was only an ad hoc body, set up to consider a particular set of issues and now disbanded. Over two years the committee built up some expertise in the area and received evidence from some 250 organisations and about 700 members of the public. Its report, however flawed, has stimulated great debate and interest. A record two million people have been spurred to sign a petition in favour of a private member's bill (albeit one opposing the Warnock majority view).

What we need now is a Super-Warnock: a permanent body to keep under view the whole range of issues in medical law and ethics. Given time such a body would be able to produce suggested codes of practice covering areas such as *in vitro* fertilisation, treatment of the young, allocation of scarce resources within the NHS and the requirements of a sensible doctrine of informed consent.

Within its own narrow field, Warnock saw the need for such an authority. Indeed the committee regarded the establishment of a new statutory authority with advisory and executive functions as 'by far the most urgent' of its recommendations.

The *raison d'etre* of its executive licensing function might well disappear if Parliament eventually bans all experiment on embryos. Nevertheless we should rescue the advisory, monitoring role and expand it to cover all the questions of medical ethics which so concern us.

It may be unfashionable to suggest new quangos but very occasionally this is just what is required. A permanent advisory committee would fulfil a need which various forms of surrogate quangohood (such as the courts, administrative fiats and ad hoc committees) cannot satisfactorily meet.

Who would oppose such a body? The government would no doubt baulk at large expenditure on a secretariat so the new quango might have to rely initially on the existing infrastructure of research for some of its information. Nevertheless, the government seems ready to accept the principle behind Warnock's proposed authority.

The medical establishment might be tempted to oppose the quango but any legitimacy in that position has been undermined by their reluctant approval of Warnock's licensing body. Doctors and researchers would have accepted that as the price for public acquiescence in their experiments. The public, however, may seize on that concession, while refusing to allow experiments, in order to create a more general review body which would work in everyone's interests, helping patients and doctors alike by extensive and expert consideration of their ethical dilemmas.

What would the new quango do? Ignoring the specific references to *in vitro* fertilisation, Warnock's explanation is a good one: 'We believe it should issue general guidance, to those working in the field, on good practice ... and on the types of research which ... it finds broadly ethically acceptable. It should also offer advice to Government on specific issues as they arise, and be available to Ministers to consult for specific guidance. As part of its responsibility to protect the public interest, it should publish and present to Parliament, an Annual Report'.

Who would be on the committee? Warnock again has the answer. 'The new body will need access to expert medical and scientific advice. We would therefore envisage a significant representation of scientific and medical interests among the membership. It would also need to have members experienced in the organisation and provision of services. However, this is not exclusively or even primarily, a medical or scientific body. It is concerned essentially with broader matters and with the protection of the public interest. If the public is to have confidence that this is an independent body, which is not to be unduly influenced by sectional interests, its membership must be wide-ranging and in particular the lay interests should be well represented.' Within the term 'lay', I would include experts in medical law and ethics.

Until recently the USA had such a quango – the inelegantly titled but otherwise admirable President's Commission for the

Study of Ethical Problems in Medicine and Biomedical and Behavioral Research. Building on that model we could surely construct an institution which was able to tackle the important task of establishing codes of practice on medical ethics in a systematic and informed way. Above all, we need to have guidelines *before* doctors and researchers face the moral dilemmas directly and this is an area where, as we have seen, 'both medical science and opinion within society may advance with startling rapidity'. Although much of the Warnock report is rightly being criticised, the committee did have the beginnings of a good idea in recommending an advisory body. That suggestion should be developed. It would be a tragedy if the embryo of a much-needed innovation is thrown out with the Warnock bath water.

Notes and references

1 Department of Health and Social Security. Report of the Committee of Inquiry into Human Fertilisation and Embryology. Cmnd 9314 (Chairman: Dame Mary Warnock) London, HMSO, 1984, reprinted with additional material by Mary Warnock as A question of life: the Warnock report on human fertilisation and embryology, Oxford, Basil Blackwell, 1985. The latter is an odd mixture, with one chapter by Mary Warnock sandwiched between her original letter to the government and the original Foreword, and her second contribution appearing between the Dissents and the Appendix. Be warned: these new chapters are merely Mary Warnock's personal views, not part of the report proper. The new pink cover seems more attractive than the official blue of the original. The new title seems ironic to critics of the report as the report does not attempt to answer directly the question of when life begins.

2 See 1 above: page ii in the HMSO version; page iv in the Blackwell version.

3 See 1 above: page 95 in the HMSO version; page 101 in the Blackwell version.

4 Catholic Bishops' Joint Committee on Bio-Ethical Issues. Report. Godalming, Catholic Media Office, paragraph 10. Copies are obtainable from the Publications Department, Ashtead Lane, Godalming, Surrey GU7 1ST.

5 See 1 above, paragraph 2.11.

6 See 1 above, paragraph 2.5.

7 See 1 above, paragraph 2.9.

8 See 1 above, pages 80 and 82 in either version.

9 See 1 above, paragraphs 12.2 and 12.3.

> 12.2 A test in which human sperm may fertilise hamster eggs is already used in the investigation of male subfertility. Men whose sperm will fertilise a specially treated hamster egg may eventually father a child, whereas those whose sperm will not are probably infertile. Although in the hamster test any resulting embryo does not develop beyond the two cell stage, it is possible that other similar forms of trans-species fertilisation tests could be developed. Unlike the hamster test, such tests might result in an embryo which might develop for a considerable period of time. Both the hamster tests and the possibility of other trans-species fertilisations, carried out either diagnostically or as part of a research project, have caused public concern about the prospect of developing hybrid half-human creatures.
>
> 12.3 We take the view that trans-species fertilisation when undertaken as part of a recognised programme for alleviating infertility, or in the assessment or diagnosis of subfertility, is an acceptable procedure, subject to certain safeguards. Since the object is to assess fertilising capacity, we see no reason why any resultant embryo should be allowed to survive beyond the two cell stage. We recommend that where trans-species fertilisation is used as part of a recognised programme for alleviating infertility or in the assessment or diagnosis of subfertility it should be subject to licence and that a condition of granting such a licence should be that the development of any resultant hybrid should be terminated at the two cell stage. Any unlicensed use of trans-species fertilisation involving human gametes should be a criminal offence.

10 See, for example, Ian Kennedy (1984/5) 34 King's Counsel 21 at page 28.

11 See 1 above, Chapter 11 and Dissents B and C. See Ian Kennedy (1984/5) 34 King's Counsel 21 for everything which needs to be said.

12 See 1 above, Chapter 8 and Dissent A.

13 See 1 above, paragraph 11.22, Dissents B and C.

14 For my immediate reactions to the Warnock report see the Catholic Herald, 27 July 1984, page 3. Also see: Warnock, law and morality. New Society, 14 February 1985, pages 263–264 for my further observations.

PERSONS, KINDS AND CAPACITIES
Keith Ward

Most people who work in medical health care are probably not particularly interested in rather abstract philosophical questions. Quite understandably, they wish to get on with the job of coping with sickness and injury. However, philosophical problems, always lying below the surface, obtrude more clamorously as medical technology advances. Health care workers are faced with ethical questions about forms of treatment, the termination or prolongation of life and the limits of medical research, in an increasing number of situations. Nowhere is this more apparent than in that group of issues which formed the subject matter of the Warnock committee of enquiry into human fertilisation and embryology. Even though the committee itself tried to avoid raising the deepest philosophical issues overtly, they were not able to avoid assuming some provisional position. In dealing with the subjects of human sexuality, personhood and procreation, they were touching on some of the deepest feelings human beings are prone to, and it is hardly surprising that the issues raised continue to be matters of lively dispute.

When a clarification of moral issues is asked for, we seek to see whether general principles can be formulated explicitly which we are prepared to accept, and which will apply to all relevantly similar cases without giving rise to consequences which we regard as undesirable. We seek for principles which will be rationally defensible, without necessarily being overwhelmingly strong. And we seek to be aware of all relevant objections and alternatives, so that we may be reasonably sure that we have considered as many aspects of the case as possible. In the case of the topics covered by the Warnock committee, it is clear that there are very basic disputes which do not seem to be resolvable. This means that there is not going to be an articulation of the issues and an adjudication on the weight of the various principles involved, which will be agreed by all informed moralists. What we will get is an articulation of various moral viewpoints which might be adopted, and of the even more basic philosophical suppositions which underlie the adoption of these viewpoints.

It is important to recognise at the outset, however, that this does not mean that we simply say, 'Let everyone make up his or her own mind according to purely personal choice'. Immediately, that would be to beg the question in favour of one viewpoint insofar as it gives a very high value to personal decision-making in ethics, and to the value of autonomy. What we may hope to see more clearly are the bases of our own moral outlook, the methods of ethical decision-making appropriate to it, and the strengths both of the arguments for it and of the objections to it. Disagreements will not always be resolved. The value of the exercise is largely clarity about one's own view; perhaps even in forming it clearly for the first time, and in being able to cope more sensitively with other views, discerning their different roots.

My aim is to exhibit two fairly well-defined moral traditions of thought which lead to very different conclusions with regard to many issues in embryology and human fertilisation. I will not seek to argue for one against the other; nor do I suggest that these are the only approaches one may adopt. But the two traditions I have selected seem to me to be very important ones, both well represented in Western societies at least. And the issues they raise lead us to consider very basic questions of outlook and methodology. I do not want to give these traditions artificial names, or to suggest that they are monolithic and opposed blocks of thought. But it may be helpful if I mention two people who have written on these themes, one from each tradition. The first is Oliver O'Donovan, Regius Professor of Moral Theology in the University of Oxford, whose book, *Begotten or Made?*, covers the main ethical issues of the Warnock committee in a brief but penetrating compass.[1] The second is Peter Singer, who has written many books and papers on these topics, but whose book *Practical Ethics* gives perhaps the best overall view of his approach to ethical issues.[2]

As the focus of discussion I will take what are perhaps the most fundamental questions raised by the Warnock report: what is a human life? And when may it be said to begin? If we are considering new, and to some extent artificial, methods of procreating human life, or possible experiment on human embryos, both these questions need to be answered. But the two traditions I have mentioned may begin to differ already on whether they can be answered, or on how to go about answering them. For the one tradition, there is a correct answer to be had, and one's moral decisions will follow naturally from the answer one gives. But for the other tradition, there may be no answer at all, or only one which is a matter of definition or convention.

Of course, both would accept that we know, in ordinary life, what a human being is, at least in standard cases. A human being can be defined biologically as possessing 46 chromosomes (normally), as a primate with a well-developed cortex, and so on. And such a being certainly begins to exist at some time, however vaguely specified. Some sort of answer can be given to the questions, then. The difficulties begin to arise when we try to be more precise, and when we ask what exactly turns on the answer we give. The reason we want an answer to the questions is that we want to know how we should treat entities which are human, or putatively human. Should we, for example, be prohibited from terminating the life of such a being? Or have we even a duty to provide for its well-being, in defined circumstances? To put it in one well-worn way, at what point are we going to ascribe human rights – at least, the rights to life and freedom from interference which causes harm – to some entity?

English law has traditionally taken the view that a person can have rights only after birth, though there is no reason why this tradition should continue to be unchanged if circumstances give cause for change, as some think they do. So a reasonable *prima facie* view would seem to be that a human life is the life of a member of the human species, and that it begins at birth. That is the view taken by Sir Immanuel Jacobovits, who holds a human life begins when the head or greater part of the body has emerged from the birth canal[3], and its end is at the cessation of respiration and blood circulation when not artificially prolonged. A human being is, under these conditions, anything born of a human mother. It is not only irrelevant, it is quite wrong to seek for further criteria by which people may be entitled to human rights, or to respect as human persons.

Within those limits, he holds, the worth of each human being is infinite, and in a twofold sense. First, no one human being is more valuable than any other, since all are infinite, and infinites cannot be compared. Second, each moment of every human life is of the same value, since the infinite is not divisible. We cannot put a limited economic value on any part of any human life, or compare different parts of qualities of human life with one another, since all have equal – infinite – value. It follows from this that we are to preserve human life at any cost, and that there is a total gap between the worth ascribed to humans and to other animals.

It may be thought a mere cavil to point out that infinites can in fact be divided; that, at least since the time of Cantor, they have been ordered into larger and smaller and can be compared by various sophisticated mathematical techniques. For the real bone of contention here is the claim that the worth of each human life is absolutely unlimited. That seems a completely unworkable principle, when surgeons do have to compare human lives, and decide, for example, which people should receive kidney dialysis. They therefore have to use some criteria of selection. And there comes a point where most doctors will hold that the expense of keeping a terminally ill person alive in great pain for a few more moments is not worth it; and thus they will judge that such moments of pain are not of unlimited value. That, of course, is a judgement of value, not of fact, and one can see very clearly why the Chief Rabbi maintains his view, difficult though it may appear. For once we start comparing human beings for value, we may seem to be set on the way to selection procedures which are still too reminiscent of Nazi Germany to be comfortably accepted.

However, if we ignore the value-judgement for a while, it is not difficult to see problems with the *prima facie* view of human life upon which it is based; or, to be more exact, with the connection between that view and the ethical capital which is made of it. For why should we value members of the human species so highly? We can decide to do so if we wish; but is our decision a reasonable and defensible one? Can we defend subscribing to a principle which says, 'Value entity x because it is a member of species y?' The trouble is that the reason offered for valuing x does not seem to be morally relevant. Why should we value members of species y more than members of species z? If we know nothing further about the species in question, there seems to be no distinguishing factor which would make a difference of treatment rational. If y was a particularly rare species, that might be a good reason for treating it specially. But then we are adding another reason, not just species-membership.

Philosophers have not been slow to point this out, and to protest at 'speciesism' as an indefensible preference for one's own species, simply on the grounds that it is the species one happens to be a member of. Of course, it may be argued that membership of a species is a relevant reason for treating another member preferentially. The parallel case would be that of treating members of one's own family preferentially just because they are members of your family. Many of the obligations and duties we come to have do depend upon contingencies of birth and circumstance, and perhaps it would be defensible to favour one's own species over others. However, the thought leaves us a little uneasy; for, while it may be acceptable to have special responsibility for members of your own family, it does not seem right to give them preference for jobs or exemption from criminal procedures. Considerations of group-membership cannot override considerations of justice. And, in formulating a moral principle, we feel the need to ascend to a more impartial viewpoint if possible in order to frame a principle that could be accepted by any rational being, whatever position such a being is in. Insofar as our principles are connected with justice, then we cannot accept the fact of species-membership alone as a good reason for preferential treatment.

Where justice is in question, we need to provide some independent justification for regarding members of the human species with special consideration. The religious believer may say that God has commanded us to do so, and God's commands are not to be questioned. But, while on matters such as the eating of certain kinds of food God may make an otherwise morally neutral matter a matter of obligation, it is hard to suppose that he might turn wrong into right. Even God's command cannot make it right to respect humans infinitely more than animals, if it would otherwise be wrong to do so. Also, we might think that even God would have reason for issuing such a command; and it may be possible for us to think of that reason.

Accordingly, philosophers have sought to make explicit what it is about the human species that makes it worthy of special consideration. What they have usually done is to list certain features, the possession of which would qualify a subject for special consideration. These features are likely to include such things as: self-awareness; the sense of an individually continuous existence over time; the capacity for awareness of God; creative membership of a cultural community. There may be dispute about specific features, but the concern is to discover and state what it is that is distinctive about human life, in paradigm cases, that may lead us to value it, or may lead any rational being to value it over the lives of other animals. There will be general agreement that the distinctive features are connected centrally with rationality and the capacity to put a value on things and pursue them freely and responsibly.

The problem with this approach is, that once we have set out a list of relevantly distinctive features, we have already in principle separated the properties from their human subjects. That is, once we have decided what the relevant set of features is, we can prescribe the general rule that anything possessing those features, or at least a reasonable sub-set of them, is worthy of special respect. Conversely, anything not possessing them is something we are not obliged to respect in the same way. This is the point at which the Chief Rabbi might reasonably begin to worry. For it seems that we can no longer concentrate attention on the human species alone. We have a list of features, which might be called features distinctive of personhood. These features may well not be limited to human beings. For example, it is quite possible that there are extra-terrestrial beings who are certainly not human, but which may possess all these features in an eminent degree. So we find that we are not respecting human life as such; but only insofar as it exhibits personal features which may be shared by many other species.

The real problem, however, is that there are many members of the human species who do not possess these features – notably young babies, severely mentally handicapped people and people suffering from such things as senile dementia. Depending on how narrowly personal features are defined, it may turn out that whole classes of human beings simply do not qualify for that special respect which we feel appropriate to persons. And that is where uneasy memories of the euthanasia policies of the Third Reich begin to stir. Such stirrings are not helped when utilitarian philosophers like R G Frey, of Liverpool University, say that brain-damaged babies may be experimented on just as animals are, since they are not properly speaking persons.[4]

It has become almost commonplace among philosophers concerned with medical ethics to distinguish between humans and persons, and to say that the proper object of our moral concern is not humans, but persons. Thus the question with which I began should now be: what is a personal life not what is a human life? We are to ask when personhood begins, not when human life begins. This changes the nature of the questions quite radically. Two rather extreme, but by no means impossible, cases may help to make the point.

If what we value is rational awareness, then we will find that some very intelligent chimpanzees will be more valuable than some brain-damaged babies. And so we might find ourselves in the position of being able to justify killing mentally handicapped babies, who need a grave and difficult operation to survive, so that their sound internal organs may be transplanted into intelligent chimpanzees. There seems to be something wrong with this, but it is very hard to say what it is. Again, if personhood requires some degree of rational awareness and moral responsibility, many people would place the beginning of personhood a number of years after birth, even in the case of normal humans. So, whatever we thought about infanticide, it would not constitute killing a person, and would be more like killing a primate of some other species. Again, this seems counter-intuitive, but is very hard to counter in terms of the arguments deployed.

I began with the suggestion that human life is simply membership of the human species, and begins at birth. The objection to this view is that, while it has *prima facie* plausibility, it is not able to give a morally relevant basis for treating humans with special moral concern. So attention comes to be focused on personhood, and we end with the suggestion that some humans, though not all, are persons, and that personhood begins with the onset of rational awareness. It is at this point that the two traditions I am concerned with begin to exhibit their differences. For the first tradition, it is largely a matter of convention what specific attributes are allocated to personhood; but at least it must lie in the presence of certain qualities. These features, however, may be manifold, imprecise and intensively continuous. That is, there may be no individual features which are either necessary or sufficient for personhood; rather, a range of features may exist, the possession of some of which may suffice for ascription of personhood. These features need not be precisely describable – the Platonic quest for exhaustive definition may be inherently misleading, and it may be better to rely on a total grasp of many overlapping characteristics. The features may not be distinct and discontinuous, as if at one moment they do not exist and at the succeeding moment they do. Rather, like the beginning of a thunderstorm, there may be a continuous process, at the beginning of which there is not a storm and at the end of which there certainly is one. Yet there is no specific moment at which the thunderstorm begins. It builds up continuously over a period of time. So personhood may build up over a period of time. It is not lacking one moment and present the next; no definite line for its beginning can be drawn.

For this tradition we may know what the central cases of personhood are, and what things are clearly not persons. But there will be a large grey area – not of things which are either persons or not, though we cannot tell which, but of things which are ambiguously persons, because as a matter of fact they do not quite fit into our conceptual definitions. In this tradition, a rule prohibiting the killing or harming of persons will not automatically extend to the grey areas. Since they are admitted to be grey, the most likely procedure is that the rule will be applied weakly at early stages in the person-forming process, and progressively more strongly as the process progresses. That is, the reasons for not killing or harming need to get progressively stronger as entities approach more and more nearly to being fully-fledged persons. The basis of this approach is that persons are to be recognised, with the qualifications made above, by the presence of actual properties, whether behavioural or mental or both.

For the second tradition, personhood is not to be ascribed or assessed in terms of the presence of an actual set of distinctive properties. What is of more fundamental importance is the existence of a substance, *hypostasis* or subject, which begins to be at a discrete point of time, which continues to have a distinctive history, receiving and losing properties continually, and which ends as discretely as it began, perhaps long after its most distinctive properties have ceased to be evident. In this view, the world is seen to consist of substances falling into various natural kinds, which possess specific potentialities for development proper to the kinds of thing in question. Each entity falls into some natural kind or class of thing; and it is proper to that class to develop towards a certain end or natural realisation. This view clearly bears the marks of an Aristotelian origin. It thinks of the world not as a valueless, purposeless and morally neutral mechanism, but as a realm of moral value and purpose. Things in nature have inherent values and purposes which lie in the realisation of their distinctive potentialities. Thus a human person will be a kind of substance which has, in its inherent constitution, the potentiality for realising the distinctive qualities of human personhood.

There are two elements in this tradition which are almost entirely lacking in the other. One is that entities are seen not merely in terms of the properties which they actually possess, but in terms of the possession of a nature which is properly realised in certain properties, but which may not be realised because of some impediment, frustration or handicap. A person may be said to exist when that nature begins to be, however potential or as yet unrealised its nature may be. The second element is that human persons are not just particular cases of a general category of persons, or rational agents in the abstract. Humans are particular kinds of persons, embodied in specific forms of sexuality, corporeality and community. There may well be persons who are asexual, whose bodily forms are very different from the human and who do not live in communities. There is no need to deny that they are persons. But to be a human person is not just to be a person contingently or peripherally associated with a certain bodily form, related to others in many physical ways. It is to be a human agent which displays personal qualities in its own proper form.

It can readily be seen how this general view will govern attitudes to questions of personhood and human life. We will not only be concerned with the ascertainable presence of properties displaying rational agency. We will primarily be concerned with the coming into being of an entity of a unique kind, which possesses the potentiality for the realisation of characteristically human qualities of personhood. The point is not that human personhood is to be valued more highly than possible forms of non-human personhood just because it is human; although it is true that one should respect all forms of rational agency, however they are embodied. The point is rather that the quality of personhood cannot be separated from the property of being human, in the case of human beings – any more than the property of being male or female can be separated from the property of being human. The object of our moral concern, in other words, is not persons who happen to be human, but human beings who have the potentiality, proper to their kind, of realising personal qualities.

This is, of course, a crucial point when the question of babies, the mentally subnormal and early embryos is under discussion. If you are looking for the presence of personhood in things which happen to be human beings, you will not find it in these human beings, or will only find it ambiguously present. Whereas if you are looking for entities which belong to a class to which it is proper to exhibit personal qualities under suitable conditions, then all these human beings are such entities, which have either not yet developed or which have been frustrated in their development by disease or impediment. It may well be held that we owe to handicapped members of a certain class a greater degree of care than we do to normally developed members of that class. This would be the moral value of care for the weak or of compassion, and in that case we would value handicapped members of a species more highly than non-handicapped members, not less.

Suppose, from this point of view, we look back at the case of the very intelligent chimpanzee and the mentally handicapped child – or, even more to the point, the human foetus, quite unconscious, which can be killed to provide organs for subsequent transplant. It will still be true that the chimp scores more highly than the human on every test for mental capacity, and thus may seem to be more of a person. But what is overlooked is that the chimp is an adult of a certain sort; it is an outstanding example of its species in full flower. The foetus, on the other hand, is a young and undeveloped individual of a different sort. It has yet to develop nearly all of its powers, and we can hardly tell what sort of thing it truly is just by looking at it. Most of its nature as yet consists in unrealised dispositions, and to describe it properly we must say that it is a young human, not that it is an entity with no sentience or rationality. We do pay regard to the future in deciding what a thing is; often, the fact that it is not yet something gives an added importance to the way we think of it. Compare how children are often saved first in emergencies; we have in mind that children have their lives before them. Their actual state of value is no doubt less than that of many adults, but they have a far greater potential value. Moreover, we do not usually stop to calculate the possible value of the child's later life, as compared with that of some adult now. Rather, we give a distinctive worth to the potentiality of the child to develop its own life, however much or little we may value it later. We say the adult has had a chance to develop its capacities; the child has not. So we give a higher priority, other things being equal, to the child – that is, to the capacity for development. We thus appear to be taking as a moral axiom that a personal being should have the chance to realise its nature, at least to a reasonable degree.

This idea of self-realisation or development of an individual nature by individual choice and action, and the consequent realisation of a unique pattern of experience is, the second tradition will say, what chiefly distinguishes persons from mere receptors of pain and pleasure. Persons can build upon their experiences, forming an experience unique in shape and pattern, contributing distinctive personal actions to the world which manifest their nature and what they have made of it by their relatively free decisions. It is the realisation of such capacities which leads us to ascribe a special worth to persons. And it leads us to give some priority to allowing beings to develop such capacities, if they can.

Some, at least, of the higher mammals may have moral capacities and emotions. Nevertheless, it would be silly to view them as full and proper partners in a moral community; to give them a say in decision-making and goal setting: to ask them to make hard moral decisions or to decide their own way of life. It is not proper to their natures to be included fully as members of a rational and moral cultural community, even though they may exhibit many desirable and valuable capacities of their own. The fact remains that we would not call a chimp handicapped if it could not stand for Parliament; whereas we would call an adult human being handicapped if he or she lacked the mental ability to do so. Such people – and of course there are many of them – lack something that is not only a human good, but that is proper to human nature. If we can speak of human nature as that set of dispositions and capacities which belongs to members of our moral community, then we can find many individuals who lack many of these dispositions. They are more adequately described as persons who lack something proper to them, than as simply non-persons. Yet even chimps can be truly called less than fully personal, insofar as they cannot participate in a moral and rational community. Accordingly, a high value may be given to undeveloped and handicapped humans, just because they belong to a kind to which it is proper to exhibit personal qualities.

But is it a morally relevant reason for treating x in a certain way that it belongs to a class with properties a, b, c.., even though x itself will never exhibit those properties? Extreme, but quite frequent, cases which make this point clearly are the severely mentally handicapped babies who will inevitably die within a few weeks. These babies, it may be confessed, belong to the class of human persons, with the properties of responsible decision-making and so on. But they themselves will never even come near to possessing such properties, so why should their class-membership be morally relevant? Why may they not be treated as organisms which will never develop a degree of awareness greater than that of some of the higher mammals, if that?

Here again, the basic difference of view with which I am concerned comes to the fore. Can we adequately say what an individual is simply in terms of its actual possession of certain properties? We certainly cannot do so if all we are thinking of is the possession of properties at some particular time. For at any given time, humans are actualising very few of their distintive capacities. A sleeping woman cannot be adequately described solely in terms of the properties she actually exhibits during deep sleep. But we may extend our view to the whole course of a person's life, and say that we can describe the person in terms of all the actualised properties in the course of that life. Then, the dying baby can be said to be the sum of its actual properties during its short life.

One difficulty here is that we will not be able to say what anything is until it has ceased to exist. Perhaps we are to make a guess at its probable course of life, and describe it accordingly? Yet there is something unsatisfactory about describing a person solely in terms of her actual performances, without referring to what she could have done, to capacities she may have had, but never realised. It is certainly a highly relevant fact about a person that she could have been a great violinist, but chose to look after her aged parents instead. So, in giving a morally relevant description of a person, we need to mention what she could or might have done, and not just all that she did.

Again, there is a distinction between the failure to exercise some capacity which a person actually has, and the lack of that capacity. I can properly say that I am a good swimmer, that I have the capacity to swim, even though I am not swimming at the moment. I have swum before, and will again; it is characteristic of me to swim; but I do not have to be doing it all the time. Nevertheless, before I had ever swum or even learned to swim, when I was so young that I had not even developed the ability to swim, it would have been false for me to say, 'I am a good swimmer'. Could I have said that I had the capacity for swimming, as yet unrealised? The difference is that the swimmer who is not at the moment swimming possesses all the necessary conditions for swimming, as far as his skills are concerned, but is not exercising his capacities. Whereas the baby has not yet developed a skill, and so lacks some necessary conditions for swimming. The baby will be said not to have any capacity as yet to exercise.

This is certainly a relevant difference. In an analogous case, we may say that a person in deep sleep is not exercising any rational skills. But we would not say that the person does not exist. For we can say that there is some subject of consciousness which has many memories, developed skills and so on, and which will exercise them when it awakes, even though it is dormant at present. But an early embryo which has not yet developed a brain, and so has not yet achieved one of the important necessary conditions for consciousness, does not yet possess any rational skills, either active or dormant.

Thus we might choose to describe a person, not only in terms of occurrent qualities which they possess, but in terms of dispositions, whether long or short term, which they exhibit. And we can sensibly say that a given being, at a given time, may possess a nature which actually has many dispositional properties. It is important to note that this account does not reduce dispositional properties merely to conjunctions of hypotheticals, such as, 'If I push her, she will run', and so on. Rather, it admits that there is an actual causal basis present in the agent, which generates sequences of hypotheticals on appropriate occasions. This actual basis of dispositions will contain many dispositional properties which are never in fact realised; so it will enable us to speak counterfactually of what a person is – to say not only what a person will do but of what that person might have done or could have done.

The admission of such a distinction immediately leads us to regard class-membership as an important component of any adequate description of an individual. For, if a description of an individual needs to incorporate statements about dispositional properties which will never in fact be realised, it follows that we cannot correctly describe that individual solely in terms of its actually and individually realised properties. We have to describe it also in terms of dispositional properties, the presence of which may only be inferred from the fact that other members of the class realise such properties. To take a very simple example, it would be correct to say of an adult human being that she has the ability to learn a foreign language, even if she will never do so, for such abilities are proper to her class (the class of adult humans) where there is no impediment. In other words, it is a reason for treating x in a certain way that it belongs to a class with properties a, b, c. ., even though x itself may never exhibit those properties. One may ascribe dispositional properties to an individual on the ground that members of the class to which it belongs characteristically possess such properties.

However, we still have the problem of young and undeveloped members of classes; members who will come to possess the dispositional properties proper to their class but who cannot yet be said to possess them. It must immediately be noted that there are an enormous number of such individuals. Probably all human beings for some years after birth have not yet developed the dispositional capacities for responsible and rationally autonomous thought. In fact, the psychologist Kohlberg at one point mentioned the disquieting statistic that, according to his investigations into the development of fully autonomous moral thinking in children, only six per cent of his samples ever developed such thought at all.[5] The spectre of biological elitism does indeed begin to loom large if only six per cent of human beings will possess fully personal dispositional properties. What of the rest of us? Do we deserve a lower degree of moral respect?

It is not obvious that we should only morally respect an individual who actually possesses those dispositional properties which we value most highly. The problems of such an approach are very great. One is the familiar philosophers' problem of whether we are justified in ascribing rational freedom (for instance) to people on more than a few rare occasions, or to more than a few rare individuals. Reputable philosophers like C A Campbell have held that occasions of truly free choice are very rare, and that perhaps most people only have one such experience in the whole of their lives. More broadly, there are serious doubts about the extent to which individuals possess such capacities; and there is no clear way of resolving such doubts, since the properties in question are so recondite and difficult to discern. We can proceed, of course, on a 'benefit of the doubt' basis, and ascribe such properties to all adults. But again we must accept that we are not, strictly speaking, judging individuals in isolation, in and for themselves, but as members of classes. If that is so, why should we limit ourselves to adult members of classes, since we value even adults largely for their potential, for what they may later become, by their own decisions?

The argument from 'potential' is a difficult one. For some philosophers, to say that x is a potential y is to say no more or less than that all or most xs tend to turn into, or to be contiguously succeeded by, ys. On that account, there is absolutely no reason why an x should be treated in the same way as a y. An x must, in short, be treated simply as an x. But, since it is one of the causal conditions for the coming-into-existence of a y, we may be concerned for it if, and only if, we want to bring about a y.

In the case of procreation, a particular sperm and an ovum may be causal conditions of the genesis of a person, but there is no reason to treat them with special respect just because of that, or with any respect at all. We can throw them down the sink, experiment on them or do whatever we like with them. However, if it so happens that we particularly want to bring a new person into existence, we will then treat the sperm and ovum with special care – but only because they are instrumental means to effecting what we want. They are deserving of no respect in themselves; we value them only if and insofar as we wish to procreate a person. Now in the first moral tradition, an early embryo is in fact in exactly the same position as the sperm and ovum just before fusion. It deserves no respect in itself; we can do what we want with it. If we happen to want to bring a person into existence, we use the embryo as a causal means to do so.

The second moral tradition which I am concerned to expound takes a very different view. At some point, it will hold, an entity comes into being which belongs to the class of entities to which it is proper to possess those dispositional properties which are constitutive of human personhood. It is therefore a vitally important matter to determine when such an entity begins to be. For that entity will possess, potentially, all those properties which characterise persons. That is to say, the entity, if allowed to develop naturally, will properly come to possess those properties.

Now it is to be noted that both traditions profess respect for persons, on the basis of certain distinctive properties which persons characteristically possess. There is, I am assuming, no dispute so far. But there is a dispute about what a person is, and how it may properly be characterised. For one view, a person must be in possession of certain capacities before it is a proper object of respect. For the other view, a person is essentially a subject which has a distinctive nature, which is realised in the fruition of certain properties but which is not exhausted by them; which in fact always transcends any descriptive set of properties and which is a locus of subjectivity set within the material world. In this respect, the dispute is between a view of persons as objects among others, which are proper matters for scientific investigation and control; and a view of persons as irreducible subjects, setting limits to control and experiment, and never wholly categorisable in objective or descriptive terminology.

In another respect, one view sees persons as primarily bundles or complexes of properties, of pleasure and pain, or of specific mental states. The other view sees persons primarily as underlying subjects, which indeed possess characteristic sets of properties and enjoy various mental states, but which are not reducible to such properties and states and which possess a unique, largely hidden reality. For the first view, talk of potential properties of persons comes down to talk of the properties they might in future exhibit, though they do not do so now. It is useless to speak of potentialities as though they were in some sense actually existent. So we can only consider the present reality as a stage on the way to the existence of some future reality. But for the second view, the potential properties of persons are a real part of what they truly are. There is a sort of causal condition in the person which would, in suitable conditions, generate specific occurrent properties in future. Accordingly, to terminate the existence of a person is to eradicate that causal condition; it is not merely to eradicate some actual properties which are not fully personal.

It is readily seen how these two views lead to different practical conclusions in specific cases. The first view is likely to lead us to decide that unwanted and severely handicapped babies may be killed, or allowed to die without any serious effort being made to preserve their lives. Such babies will not of themselves possess any person-features; and so they are to be valued for extrinsic reasons – because parents or others want them to live or value them for some emotional reason. Where those extrinsic factors do not obtain, and where respect for human life is not going to be undermined in general, there is accordingly no reason for keeping those babies alive.

The difficulty with this view is that the principle seems to extend very readily to cases in which adult humans are not wanted or loved or valued by anyone and where their quality of life or mental capacities are very low – one thinks, for example, of city down-and-outs or of many drug-addicts and possible suicides. One may simply accept the analogy offered, and say that such people ought to be allowed to die when they are in need of expensive medical care. But we should be aware that this is the course we are set upon.

On the second view of personhood, each existent person is to be valued as one not to be harmed gratuitously, entitled to a reasonable degree of medical care. The mental capacities or states of mind of the person will not be assessed before deciding whether his or her life is to be preserved, except perhaps in those cases in which we have to choose only one of a number of persons to be treated. We will be committed to respect for personhood as such, where personhood is not to be defined in terms of occurrent properties or actual dispositional capacities, but rather in terms of the possession of a nature which would properly be realised, if there were no impediments, in a rational and reasonable existence. Moreover, it is most important to understand that, on this second view, the moral principle adopted is not seen as a mere decision. It is not a matter of just deciding to draw a line at some more or less arbitrary place. Rather, human persons are distinctive types of entity, and our moral response to them is precisely a response which is appropriate to the form of reality which they possess. The moral principle is not in some odd way deducible from a statement of the facts; it is seen as an appropriate response to the facts, when properly discerned.

The difference between the two views, then, is not just a difference of moral principles – as though each agreed about the facts, and decisions about values were optional extras which each person is free to decide upon as they choose. Such an account already adopts the first viewpoint, for which the world and human nature are morally neutral, and moral decisions are choices which we are free to make as we wish. The difference is about the nature of the facts, and it involves fundamental differences of view of the natural order and the place of human nature within it. It involves a fundamental difference in our understanding of the basis of morality. Is it a set of principles freely chosen to safeguard or implement more effectively one's desires, or is it a response to the discernment of how things truly are – a discernment in which desires will play an important part, but in which they are to be conformed to the discernment of the real, rather than be made the blind masters of a purely instrumental reason?

I am not attempting to argue for one of these views, but to articulate the nature of disagreements in this area of human nature and procreation, and to show how very deep they are. This, in turn, may help us to see the ramifications and presuppositions of the moral views we are inclined to take. And it may help us to understand the views of others. Moral analysis will not resolve the problems. But it may make the options clearer, and enable us to asses their strengths and weaknesses more fully.

The question with which I began still remains, and takes on a special urgency for proponents of the second viewpoint. Whereas for the first tradition it is a matter of decision when personhood can be said to begin and a rational decision will be made at some point in the gradual and continuous emergence of person-features in the life of an individual; for the second tradition, there is a discrete point, not to be defined in terms of the exhibition of person-features, at which a person, an entity of a kind to which it is natural to realise person-features, begins to exist. When will this point be?

Within the Christian tradition, which has constituted one main form of this second viewpoint, the morally relevant point has been seen as that at which a human soul could be said to come into existence. What was considered to be of most relevance was the fact that a person is an irreducible subject, not merely an observable object. It is a subject of experience and of agency, a sensitive and rational consciousness. It was not the case, at least in the mainstream Christian tradition, that this subject was some sort of disembodied entity which somehow comes into relation with a suitably formed body. This may be true for those Indian religious traditions which view each soul as the reincarnation of a particular ego which has had an infinite number of previous earthly existences, and so is an already well-formed character, with its karmic train of good or ill desert to be worked out in the new body. And it may be true of allegedly Cartesian dualists, for whom the soul is a distinct substance, capable of a fully personal disembodied existence. Christian theologians, generally speaking, accepted something much more like Aristotle's account, according to which the soul is the 'form' of the body. Obscure as it is, this view rejects the idea of a separate soul-entity, and insists that the subject of rational consciousness is, properly speaking, the activating principle of a particular kind of body. It comes to exist for the first time within a human body, and is its central organising principle, directing both the nutritive, sentient and rational operations of the human person. In modern terms, there comes to exist, at a certain point in the development of the central nervous system, a subject of consciousness. It is at this point that we may speak of the organism as an embodied soul; or, to put it another way, as a piece of matter so structured that it generates a subject of awareness within itself, as an emergent characteristic of its own material organisation. For Thomas Aquinas, this happened when, as he put it, the foetus was formed – that is, he thought, at about 40 days after fertilisation, in the case of males, and 90 days in the case of females.[6] Ignoring the gratuitous sexism of this guess, I think it would be fair to construe this as saying that the soul is infused into the body when the brain is formed and begins to function – which, it happens, is at about 42 days after fertilisation.

The reason for this decision about the beginning of human personhood is clear. We are concerned to find the beginning of an entity which will in due course develop rational awareness; and it seems reasonable to say that, since we are concerned about consciousness, and not only about pieces of matter, however well and complicatedly organised, it is the person as a subject of consciousness that we are really concerned with. Consciousness, it is generally agreed, does not exist before the formation of the brain; and so that seems the most rational point at which to place the beginning of the soul, the subject of consciousness. However primitive the awareness may be at first, the subject of awareness is still, from the first, a human subject of consciousness; and so must be regarded as a human person from that point. This view can, I think, make a good claim to be the traditional view of Catholic moral theologians; and it has not been officially repudiated by the magisterium of the Catholic church.[7]

Nevertheless, there are difficulties with it. The main difficulty lies in the consideration that the human person is an *embodied* subject of consciousness. If we take the full force of this consideration, we will have to admit that the characteristics of the adult person are present potentially in the genetic structure of the embryo, long before the rise of consciousness or the formation of the central nervous system. If we have agreed to speak of the genesis of an entity which will subsequently develop person-features, should we not be speaking of an entity which will subsequently develop awareness, among other things? It is, after all, the human embryo, as an entity, which develops consciousness at a certain stage; and many of the characteristics of that subject of consciousness will be governed by genetic factors which are set before any actual consciousness comes into existence.

Thus the embryo has a genetic nature which possesses all those dispositions which will result in the development of consciousness, and in the possession by that consciousness of many important traits of character and temperament, as well as more obviously physical traits such as eye-colour and height. It may seem, then, that to the extent that we think that the human being is truly one entity, an embodied self, and not an amalgam of two – a body and a mind which is connected to it – we must see the subject of consciousness as, at the same time, a subject of those physical properties which are so important to embodied persons. If it is truly the same subject we are talking about, which possesses both physical and mental properties, then it is artificial to locate the beginning of that subject at the point of the first conscious experience. It may be true that what we value about human persons is their possession of consciousness as well as their capacity for rational decision-making. But if we begin to value the subjects of rational decision-making even before they begin to make such decisions, it may well be held that we should value the subjects of consciousness before they actually become conscious. Genetic make-up does not, after all, change at neuralation; so it does not, in general, develop new capacities after the formation of the genetic mix at fertilisation.

So we may say that, even though 'ensoulment' may not occur until six weeks or so after fertilisation, at conception an entity does begin to exist to which it is proper to develop awareness at a subsequent date. It is for this reason, no doubt, that the Catholic bishops, while professing agnosticism about the time of infusion of the soul into the body (or, as we might put it, the time of the genesis of the subject of consciousness in the human being) nevertheless maintain that human life should receive protection even in its earliest stages, and thus is never a proper subject for experiment.[8] It is implausible to say that a sperm and an ovum, one centimetre apart in a glass dish, form an entity which will be a rational person – for they are as yet two entities. But when they fuse, one entity exists; and that is why fertilisation seems, on this view, to be the most appropriate discrete moment at which human personhood may be said to begin.

If we do not accept the total outlook of persons as individuals of kinds to which it is proper to develop person-features, this decision will seem odd or irrational. What feature has a three-day-old embryo got that makes it look remotely like a rational human being? And if it is cultured *in vitro*, what human persons have any love for it or desire that it should develop? Or what reason is there to fear that, if we experiment on it, our own lives or the lives of those we love might be imperilled by mad medical experimenters?

However, for the person who sees these small bundles of cells as entities of a particular kind, with their own proper, immanent teleology, questions about what they actually look like, or who loves them or desires their benefit are irrelevant to the issue, as are questions about the security or fears of other people. The only relevant question is what practical response is appropriate to entities of this kind, with the distinctive nature that they possess. And the problems that are usually brought up to throw doubt on their status cannot have the force they would have for those who see things from the other viewpoint.

For example, it is sometimes argued that a great number of

fertilised ova never could develop into recognisable human beings. They are mere masses of cells, which are usually spontaneously aborted or which never implant. These entities may have no physical organisation at all, much less a central nervous system or brain-stem. If a sperm and an ovum fuse and cell division begins yet the cells never begin to differentiate into specific functions and subsequently the cell-mass is aborted and dies, in what sense, however minimal, can that be called even a handicapped person? Again, a large number – perhaps more than 50 per cent – of early concepti are lost through natural wastage.[9] So it is asked, how can we claim that such things, of which the mothers may be unaware, have human rights in any intelligible sense?

In the first place, it must be remembered that the rights in question are the rights not to be harmed or killed. No one is suggesting that they have the right to holidays with pay. But, of course, experiment on someone, without their consent, is a form of harm. And it is generally agreed that no one may legitimately consent to being directly harmed (as opposed to taking a risk of harm which is not unreasonable).[10] Thus, if an embryo is any sort of human person, it looks as if experiment which produces direct harm or destruction is impermissible.

It will be pointed out that, in the days when infant mortality was running at more than 50 per cent of births, this was no reason for regarding babies as expendable. So the fact that so many embryos are lost by natural wastage is irrelevant to the moral issue. Those cell-masses which fail to develop are precisely that – they are human persons which fail to develop even to the earliest stages of cell-differentiation. In the case of such entities, it will seem inappropriate to keep them alive by extreme medical means – just as it is inappropriate to keep anacephalic babies alive by using scarce surgical resources. They are doubtless destined for early death; nevertheless, the double ethic of care for the weak and respect for human personhood dictates that they should not be used for forms of experimental research which cause them grievous harm for the sake of others. For this view, it is irrelevant what their actual properties are, or what their predictable course of life, as individuals, will be. The relevant moral issue is what kind of entity they are, and what the distinctive and natural properties of that kind of entity are. Only when we are clear about those things, it will be said, can we be sure of having a clear principle of respect for human beings, prohibiting all forms of interference which knowingly frustrate the natural development of their proper capacities and which will open the way to principles of selection and assessment which are potentially immoral.

This view has been well defended by the philosopher Jenny Teichman, who writes: 'In order to count as a person an individual creature need not itself be actually rational, as long as it belongs to a rational kind'.[11] Moreover, she argues, 'being a human being i.e. a human animal, is a sufficient condition of being a person'[12], since human animals are at least one natural species which belong to the very broad kind of 'personal beings'.

We are now in a position to see clearly the two different traditions which underlie the major disputes in this area. One tradition begins by thinking of classes of entity which possess various natural powers and dispositions, and adopts the moral axiom that we should not impede the realisation of these powers. We may have some duty to encourage such realisation. We should adopt an attitude of humility before the workings of the natural order, cherishing the structures which have made our lives possible, and being prepared to defer to the immanent laws of its working. We must, in other words, be prepared to a large extent to accept and value what is given to us, being committed in advance to treating all human beings as persons. We must not ourselves invent criteria for when things may or may not be fit to be called persons; or feel free to regard nature solely as a sphere of possible products and technological innovations.[13]

The other tradition rejects the concept of 'natural kinds' and of 'natural powers'. It rejects the derivation of human obligations from consideration of such natural facts. It regards nature as morally neutral and as without immanent purpose or value. Instead, it founds morality on desires, especially on the most basic and widespread desires which human beings share. It sees no virtue in accepting the structures of nature as they are. Rather, the human will is free to decide how to shape nature to its own purposes and desires. Questions of human procreation and the associated questions of how family, sexual or social life should be arranged, are simply questions of maximising human freedom, and those desires which do not tangibly harm others.[14]

In the one tradition, such questions are to be answered by asking what the nature of a human person is; what the status of the embryo is; and what the appropriate response to that sort of reality is. It will be considered to be a question of objective truth, however difficult to ascertain; and it will rely upon universal principles which are taken to be overriding and, in their basic structure, unalterable.

In the other tradition, the question of experiment on embryos is to be answered by deciding whether any basic human desires are threatened or fulfilled by experiment. This might depend on the situation, on people's actual reactions. It will therefore be resolved pragmatically, being aware that we are making a free decision. But it will be clear that embryos themselves cannot plausibly be regarded as involved in the process of decision-making, even proleptically.

Part of my purpose in writing this paper has been to set out some of the main issues underlying some of the key recommendations of the Warnock report on embryology and human fertilisation. But my primary purpose has been to show that some, at least, of the disputes are not just differences of value judgement about particular issues. Nor are they differences of decision about what to do in particular cases. Rather, they are philosophical differences about the nature of the world, the basis of moral decision-making itself, and the meaning and worth of human life, as such. In this area, at least, we can see that values are not wholly distinct from facts; that the much vaunted 'fact-value distinction' is a simplified presentation of a partial view of moral matters; and that how we see the world is often something presupposed to and determinative of particular moral decisions. The moral is not simply supervenient upon the factual, or a matter of subjective choice imposed upon agreed facts. The fundamental disagreements are about the structure of the natural order, the nature of human being; the limits (if any) on human mastery of nature, and the basis of morality. It is not surprising that it is hard to find a method of resolving them.

I have tried to expose some of the roots of the major disagreements which exist in the area of embryology, and to suggest that at least two very different ways of approaching the issue exist and are important in our historical context. I have tried to articulate these two ways, and to show how they consist of a number of closely intertwined considerations which help to constitute a total view. I have not tried to judge between them; and if I have spent more time on the 'natural kinds' tradition, it is because it is perhaps the less fashionable, in a voluntarist and technologically-oriented society. From what I have said, even in this brief space, it should be clear why the Warnock committee felt that such basic issues could not fall within its purview. But they are the issues we shall all ultimately have to face. It is only when we are clearer about these issues that we can know the basis upon which we proceed to make our own considered moral decisions in this important area.

Notes and references

1 Oliver O'Donovan. Begotten or made? Oxford, Oxford University Press, 1984.

2 Peter Singer. Practical ethics. Cambridge, Cambridge University Press, 1980.

3 Sir Immanual Jacobovits. Jewish medical ethics. Journal of Medical Ethics, 9, June 1983, pages 109–112. Also, in this volume, see page 115.

4 R G Frey. Vivisection, morals and medicine. Journal of Medical Ethics, 9, June 1983, pages 94–97.

5 L Kohlberg. Development of moral character and ideology. In: M L Hoffman (ed). Review of child development research. New York, Holt, 1964.

6 Thomas Aquinas. Summa theologiae. Blackfriars, 1964, qu 118, 2 ad 2.

7 66 Acta apostolicae sedis, 1974, page 738.

8 In vitro fertilisation: morality and public policy. Catholic Information Services, 1983, part 2, 9, note 2.

9 J O Drife. What proportion of pregnancies are spontaneously aborted? British Medical Journal, 286, 1983, page 294.

10 The Nuremberg Code (1974) and the Declaration of Helsinki (1964).
11 Jenny Teichman. The definition of person. Philosophy, April 1985, page 182.
12 See 11 above, page 184.
13 For an excellent defence of this view see: Teresa Inglesias. In vitro fertilisation: the major issues. Journal of Medical Ethics, 1, March 1984, pages 32–37.
14 This view is epitomised in the title of the book by J L Mackie, Ethics: inventing right and wrong. Harmondsworth, Penguin, 1977.

WARNOCK AND SURROGATE MOTHERHOOD: SENTIMENT OR ARGUMENT?

Shelley Roberts*

THE NATURE OF THE PROBLEM

In chapter one of the Book of Genesis, God addresses Adam and Eve with the first commandment given the human race: 'Be fruitful and multiply.'[1] In 1985, approximately one out of every six married couples in our society is unable to fulfil that commandment because of infertility.[2]

The incidence of infertility has risen noticeably in recent years and can be attributed to several factors. The increase in cases of venereal disease and of abortion, the use of certain methods of contraception, the effect of environmental pollutants and the trend towards commencing child-bearing at a later age than previously was the case, have all been cited as reducing the likelihood of successful conception.[3] At the same time, adoption, once the alternative open to childless couples, has become almost impossible. The availability of abortion and the growing social acceptability of single parenthood have left very few babies needing to be adopted.[4]

Thus, many prospective parents have been led to consider some of the more novel means of alleviating childlessness. Among these are a plethora of fertility treatments, artificial insemination by donor (AID), *in vitro* fertilisation (IVF) and, most recently, surrogate motherhood.

The term 'surrogate motherhood' has come to refer to any situation in which there is an arranged separation of the

---

* I wish to express my thanks to Professor I M Kennedy for his kindness in reading and making comments on a draft of this chapter. The responsibility for any errors remains my own. Shelley Roberts

genetic, gestational and social components of motherhood. The woman acting as surrogate agrees to give birth to a child and then to transfer its custody to the 'commissioning parents'. Such transactions are not entirely the products of modern fertilisation technology; the Bible records at least two instances in which a barren wife requested her maidservant to bear her husband's child in order to continue the family lineage.[5]

The modern form of surrogate motherhood usually employs one of the artificial fertilisation techniques, rather than resorting to an adulterous liaison, as was the case in earlier times. There are two primary varieties of surrogacy. In the first, a woman is infertile and her husband's sperm is used to inseminate artificially a second woman, the surrogate. She bears the child, then gives it up to the couple. The second method is available when a woman is fertile, but cannot carry a child to term. Her ovum is removed and fertilised *in vitro* by her husband's sperm. The embryo is then implanted in the womb of the second woman, who bears the child and gives it to the genetic parents. In each case, it is generally contemplated that the woman who acts as surrogate will receive financial compensation.

There may, of course, be permutations of both arrangements. In one example, a child could have five 'parents': the commissioning adults (a married couple, two single friends, a homosexual partnership, and so on), the sperm donor, the ovum donor and the surrogate who bears the child.

In recent times, it is the first method of surrogacy, that of artificial insemination, that has attracted most attention. This is basically because doctors involved in IVF programmes have been reluctant to accept patients requesting embryo transfer to a donor and have focused their attentions instead on married couples of which the wife is herself able to bear the child fertilised *in vitro*.

Since the late 1970s, a number of American individuals and agencies have become interested in organising surrogate transactions and have offered such services as recruiting women, screening and counselling them and arranging for their insemination on behalf of clients wishing to commission a child.

The payments collected by the agencies from the commissioning parents are divided between the surrogate and the agency.

This practice was little known in England until early 1984, when the establishment of a branch of one of the American organisations was announced. The first birth resulting from this agency's efforts took place in January 1985. For a fee of £13,000, the Surrogate Parenting Centre of Great Britain arranged, on behalf of an anonymous foreign couple, the insemination, by the husband, of a woman whom he and his wife had never met. The child born to the surrogate, Mrs Kim Cotton, was then to be handed over to the couple. The publicity arising out of this event caused the local authority in Barnet to make a 'place of safety' application as regards the infant. Such an order enables a child to be made a ward of court, and is ordinarily requested in cases where it is felt that he or she faces some form of threat in the home environment. The application was granted and Mr Justice Latey then had to determine who should have custody of the child. With no opposition from Mrs Cotton and evidence that the couple were well-suited to raise a child, the judge permitted the couple to take the child back to their home.[6]

Not surprisingly, the incident provoked a furore. One Member of Parliament referred to the arrangement as 'scandalous, sick and unnatural'.[7] The popular reaction was, in large part, one of voyeuristic curiosity. There was a certain amount of bewilderment at the motivations of the parties and especially at the mercenary detachment perceived in the surrogate. A more forceful condemnation was reserved for the agency whose American director had previously claimed she wanted 'to become the Coca-Cola of the surrogate parenting industry'.[8]

The case of Baby Cotton arose six months after the publication of the report of the Warnock Committee's Investigation into Human Fertilisation and Embryology, with its recommendations on surrogacy. This combination of events led to the hasty preparation by the government of a bill on Surrogacy Arrangements (Bill 116) which received its first reading on 1 April 1985. The Surrogacy Arrangements Bill would prohibit what it terms 'commercialised surrogacy', that is, surrogacy arranged through a paid intermediary. The bill would also ban all advertising related to surrogacy transactions.

In this paper, an attempt will be made to analyse the basis of the proposed legislation relating to surrogacy. This will be done through an examination of the influential report of the Warnock committee and a consideration of its efficacy, both in analysing the problems of surrogacy and in proposing solutions.

WARNOCK ON SURROGACY: AN INTRODUCTION

Each of the topics considered by the Warnock report was analysed within the same structural framework. First, a subject was introduced with a general explanation. Arguments for and against the practice were then enumerated. Finally, the 'Inquiry's View' was presented and explained, with (where relevant) recommended changes in the law set out.

If one turns first to this final section, the 'Inquiry's View' on surrogacy, a clear statement of disapproval emerges from the recommendations. The committee proposed a ban, accompanied by criminal sanctions, upon agencies (profit or non-profit) and other intermediaries who 'knowingly assist in the establishment of a surrogate pregnancy'. Professionals were specifically enjoined against participation.[9]

The committee did not, however, suggest that 'private' arrangements, directly negotiated between couple and surrogate, be outlawed. It seems, therefore, that in such cases, 'anything goes'. There are no restrictions on the age, marital status, sexual orientation or appropriateness for parenthood of the commissioning parent(s), nor on the woman to be hired as surrogate. Payments of any amount may be made and the parties are to be left free to negotiate the terms of their agreements. Of course, if there were any disagreement and the matter came before a court, all contracts would be declared unenforceable and disputes over custody resolved according to the best interests of the child concerned.

In order to discover why this approach was adopted for the control of surrogacy arrangements, it would seem sensible to look at the justifications outlined in the 'Inquiry's View'. Clearly, the 'Arguments against surrogacy' must have prevailed. Very few indications emerge, however, as to which amongst these arguments, presented earlier in the report, had been found by the committee to be particularly compelling. The reason offered to explain the proposed sanctions is outlined in a few phrases within a single paragraph. 'Moral and social objections' are cited. The only specific factors mentioned are the 'danger of exploitation' and the 'treatment of others as a means to one's own ends', condemned as objectionable in itself and 'positively exploitative' when done for financial interests.[10] We are left somewhat bereft of guidance as to how the committee distinguished between the various arguments advanced against surrogacy. It must therefore be assumed that all, or at least most, of these arguments were actually considered relevant and that in them lies the ground for the recommendations made in the report.

ARGUMENTS AGAINST SURROGACY

The first point stressed by the committee in its discussion of the arguments against surrogacy was 'the weight of public opinion is against the practice'.[11] This is not substantiated by any specific data, beyond a reference to 'evidence submitted to us'. Nevertheless, it may be quite reasonable to infer from the reaction to the subsequent Cotton case that there is at least a substantial degree of popular unease about surrogate motherhood.

It may be instructive at this point to examine more closely this notion of adverse public opinion which appeared to have a considerable effect upon the committee's conclusions regarding surrogacy. In other areas of the report, for example, that dealing with embryo research, to which an equally vocal segment of the population had expressed strong opposition, such reactions were, by contrast, dismissed in favour of practical exigencies, such as the 'essential' need to continue research.[12] This seems a curious descrepancy.

At least some of the confusion must stem from the explanatory Foreword to the report, a statement of the philosophy and policies of the committee. There, the reader is warned that, in the emotionally-charged areas in question, 'moral indignation or acute uneasiness' may usurp the place of argument. However, we are assured that the committee has based its own views on 'argument rather than sentiment'.

At the same time, we are told that 'moral conclusions cannot be separated from moral feelings' and are informed that the committee was 'bound to take very seriously the feelings expressed in the evidence'. How one is to determine which issues are to be analysed by argument and which decided on the basis of sentiment is not further explained, nor is any compromise or combination of the two proposed. This unfortunate confusion tends to pervade the entire document.

The conclusions of the Warnock committee on the subject of surrogate motherhood certainly suggest that a decision was made to have recourse to the criminal law in response to the concerns of public sentiment. The method chosen quite neatly reflects the subsequent public reaction to the Cotton case. Thus, the commercial agency appears as the chief menace, to be restrained by legal sanctions. The individual participants, however, are left unhindered. It seems that, although they may be engaged in distasteful or even immoral activities, these are not to be prohibited by law, as long as they are not flaunted before those whom they disturb, for example, through advertisements. The public finds surrogate motherhood unpleasant and so the law is asked to restrict those manifestations of the practice it sees as particularly unseemly.

Is this a justifiable application of the criminal law? According to the Warnock committee, the role of the law is to serve as the 'embodiment of a common moral position'.[13] Those who would accept this premiss might argue, nevertheless, that to demonstrate such a common moral position on a subject, something more than strong public feelings have to be shown. 'Common morality' is not to be equated with the vagaries of popular emotion. Immediate, instinctive reaction to a moral dilemma may exaggerate, misinterpret or overlook certain aspects of the problem. Thus, in the case of surrogate motherhood, any analysis of the role of law must first involve an examination of the specific moral arguments underlying the popular reaction and a consideration of whether these point towards any restriction upon surrogacy. If they do, then the questions arise of whether morality also dictates that such a restriction actually be imposed by law and of what form of restriction is appropriate so as to correspond to the harm perceived.

If we return to the 'Arguments against surrogacy', we find three specific points which go beyond the notion of adverse public sentiment and may help to explain it. First, it is suggested that surrogacy introduces a third party into the intimacy of the marital relationship in a protracted, intrusive and detrimental fashion. Secondly, it is argued that surrogate motherhood is potentially exploitative of or harmful to the women acting as surrogates and demeaning of women in general. Finally, it is said that the process may cause damage to the resulting children or undermine our notions of parental relationships and responsibilities.

If the Warnock committee does believe that argument should prevail over sentiment, if it is at all anxious to avoid allegations that its solution to surrogacy is simply a gesture to placate public sentiment, then it is these specific arguments against surrogacy which must be addressed. These arguments must be shown to provide suitable reasons for acting to restrain the practice and the sanctions proposed must further be justified as responding adequately to the problems identified. It is submitted that such demonstration or justification is absent from the Warnock report and that the committee has, in this respect, fallen short of its obligations. This is best demonstrated by examining in turn each of the three arguments advanced by the committee against surrogacy.

A. The three-parent family

The Warnock report states that objections to surrogacy

> ... turn essentially on the view that to introduce a third party into the process of procreation which should be confined to the loving partnership between two people, is an attack on the value of the marital relationship.[14]

The precise nature of this 'attack' was not explained, but reference was made to the section of the report dealing with 'Arguments against AID'.[15] There, some of the potential psychological threats to a stable relationship were outlined and the philosophical and moral arguments against a separation of the unitive and procreative components of marriage were also considered. The conclusion reached was that the participation in conception of a donor did not *necessarily* constitute a threat to the marital relationship. Those who found AID unacceptable could abstain; they were not, on philosophical or psychological grounds, entitled to prevent others from using AID.

The committee, contrasting surrogate motherhood and AID, stated that the two could be distinguished in that the contribution of the surrogate was 'greater, more intimate and personal'.[16] Ought this to affect the moral response or the legal treatment afforded the parties? The philosophical objection to third party intrusion is identical in both cases. While it is admitted that there may be a greater risk of psychological harm in surrogacy, it is questionable whether the possible difference is sufficient to outlaw most surrogate transactions, whilst the committee recommends that AID become organised and subsidised under the NHS.

There are two further difficulties with the analysis. The first is the factual presumption that surrogacy will lead to psychological harm and marital strain for the couple concerned. It is easily arguable that a married couple suffering despair over infertility may be psychologically helped rather than harmed by the addition of a baby born through a surrogate. The surrogate would not be interfering with, but actually enabling, procreation and thereby enhancing the relationship.

Secondly, there is the jurisprudential question of whether the law (to be specific, the criminal law) ought to interfere paternalistically in order to protect married couples from the voluntarily assumed risk of 'psychological hardship'. The implications of such an approach are somewhat daunting. Even in cases of far more blatant intrusion into the marriage, such as adultery, the criminal law is not felt to have a role to play.

Finally, even if it were accepted that surrogacy constituted an excessive intervention into the marital relationship and one that ought to be prohibited, the efficacy of the Warnock recommendations in resolving the issue might still be questioned. The elimination of commercial surrogacy would, of course, curtail the volume of the problem. However, for those couples who choose lawfully to go ahead with private arrangements, Warnock might actually encourage the marital disharmony it sought to avoid. For example, the transactions would, of necessity, be private and therefore would involve close personal contact between the surrogate and the couple. This might create a far more deleterious intrusion into the marriage than would an anonymous transaction negotiated by a competent agency.

B. The surrogate

The second major objection to the practice of surrogate motherhood raised in the report deals with the allegedly harmful effect of the procedure on the surrogate herself. There may be two types of harm suggested here. First, there is the possibility of tangible physical and psychological threats involved for the surrogates and, secondly, the threat of a more subtle distortion of societal attitudes towards the role of women and the dignity of all human beings. These can be examined in turn.

1. IS SURROGACY EXPLOITATIVE?

The possibilities for exploitation of surrogate mothers are, of course, enormous. We read, for example, of the abuses perpetrated in 'stud farms', such as one discovered in the United States, in which a group of Miami lawyers persuaded impoverished immigrant girls to be inseminated and bear children for their clients in exchange for the slum-like living conditions of the 'farm' and a little pocket money.[17]

One survey conducted by an American psychiatrist revealed that 40 per cent of the women offering themselves as surrogates were unemployed and receiving welfare benefits.[18] While it is arguable that an adult woman should be permitted to choose the means by which she alleviates her desperate financial condition, some might suggest that such a 'choice' was actually a form of coercion thereby constituting exploitation to which no valid consent could be given.

For a very poor woman, unable to find work, the sum of money offered in a surrogate transaction (usually from £6–10,000) may appear so tantalising as to overcome any caution she may otherwise exercise. Similarly, of course, the pleas of a childless sister or friend could be equally coercive. Furthermore, the dangers in pregnancy are easily minimised and the psychological risks of such an arrangement especially difficult to assess or comprehend in advance. A 'choice' made under pressure and without adequate understanding of the undoubted drawbacks may be one in which autonomy is subverted through duress. Ought the law to prohibit surrogacy on this ground? An attempt to analyse the surrogacy transaction through analogies may assist in providing an answer.

i. Surrogacy as employment
It has been suggested by some feminists that the advent of paid surrogacy has at last given recognition to the important work done by mothers and has legitimised childbearing as an occupation.[19] Certainly, the receipt of payment for tasks of hardship and risk is not *prima facie* deemed so exploitative as to render it illegal. Our country permits (even conscripts) young men to act as fighter pilots in wartime. Society recruits and the law allows miners, construction workers and trawlermen to work in occupations which may drain them of their vitality. There are specific provisions for 'danger pay' in numerous forms of employment. In at least some of these cases, the employees may have taken the jobs as a matter of last resort, unable to find work elsewhere.

To the argument that there is a social benefit attached to many high-risk occupations, childless couples would certainly argue that surrogates perform an equally noble service. Furthermore, even the 'profession' of prostitution, which many would consider both dangerous and of dubious social value, is permitted to continue, albeit under restricted conditions. Thus, if surrogacy can be classified as employment and the risks have been accepted by the women involved, it seems on one argument that the practice may not be deemed exploitative in general, or at least no more so than others permitted by law.

But is surrogate motherhood really a form of employment? Some of its features would suggest that it is not. Unlike most jobs, it does not prevent the surrogate from holding other positions contemporaneously. There are no specific tasks to perform (aside from the crucial 'passive' presence of the surrogate at the time of insemination and delivery). Furthermore, the requirements imposed upon a surrogate as a consequence of the agreement all relate to aspects of life ordinarily considered to be outside the ambit of employer–employee relations, and, if part of a contract, many might even be illegal. The surrogate is 'on duty' 24 hours a day, every day. There is no possibility of terminating the employment (without incurring criminal, or at least moral sanctions by having an abortion). The commissioning couple seeks to assert control not over work, but over aspects of personal life such as diet, medical care, sexual relations, the ingestion of alcohol and tobacco and even psychological attitude (not forming a bond with the child is one of the covenants included in some surrogacy agreements). Thus, such an agreement does not seem to be employment, as we know it, but rather something akin to slavery.

ii. Surrogacy as the disposition of a bodily organ

The law relating to the disposition or sale of human tissue has developed in a somewhat piecemeal fashion. The UK is one of the few western countries in which there are no express statutory provisions against commercial dealings in parts of the body; nevertheless, trade in bodily organs is generally considered contrary to public policy.[20] The probable exceptions are the sale of blood and sperm. In practice, of course, there are few instances of the sale of blood, but sperm donors regularly receive about £10 for their services. By analogy, ovum donation might also be paid for. American law in this area has established that the payment is given not in respect of the sale of biological material but, rather, for the provision of a service.[21]

If it is accepted that a woman may quite lawfully be compensated for the time and effort given in donating her ova, may she then also lease her womb for reward? This would seem a quite logical extension of the service contract notion. Furthermore, if we find it completely acceptable to think of a woman offering her physical and mental strength to serve as a nurse in the care of a newborn baby, why not simply extend the idea backward in time and allow for what can be called pre-natal nannies?

The answer may lie in the nature of what surrogacy involves. It is a complete, albeit temporary, disposal of part of one's body. It is arguable that there ought to be a distinction made between body material that can be sold, tissue that can only be donated and organs that may not even be given away. The law is clear as regards the last group. There are certain organs without which a person cannot survive, such as the heart and liver. Their removal cannot be rendered permissible by consent and would be considered a crime. Were it technically possible, we would also baulk at the donation of hands or feet, even though these are not indispensable to life.

The first category would arguably comprise renewable material, such as blood and sperm, as regards which the extraction process is relatively harmless and painless. This leaves the intermediate group, where donation is allowed, but commercialisation is arguably contrary to public policy. In this category might be found such body tissue as kidneys, skin and bone marrow.

Can the sale of a womb, or rather its nine-month lease, be categorised within one of these headings? As regards the matter of nine months, it seems to make little difference to distinguish between permanent and temporary dispositions of tissue. We would disallow the lease of a heart on the same grounds that we forbid its outright sale or donation. Similarly, we would probably allow a kidney to be borrowed temporarily, but question the commercial lending of the organ for reward, were such a procedure medically feasible. If the functioning capacities of these organs could be borrowed without actual removal from the body, it is suggested that this would make no difference to the analysis.

What, then, of surrogacy? Surrogate motherhood contemplates the temporary borrowing of a womb's physiological capabilities, such that they cannot be used by the woman in whose body the womb is situated, but it does not involve the removal of the organ. Such a disposition of the womb would not be so severe as to result in death or serious impairment, provided all went well. Thus, borrowing a womb does not fall into the third category, which would make it always unlawful. The first category of tissue use, however, seems equally inappropriate, as surrogacy could certainly not be characterised as a harmless or painless procedure. Thus, it seems that the intermediate position is indicated. Society will permit a gratuitous donation, but ought to condemn the sale, lease, or other exchange of the womb for money.

2. WOMEN AS MACHINES

No matter which of the above analogies is advocated, those who regard the practice of payment for childbearing as a recognition of the importance of this role of women may well have overlooked a more worrisome aspect of the transactions involved. Instead of acknowledging the worth of women, surrogacy seems more likely to reduce them to the long-despised position of child-bearing machines. The Warnock report detected this problem and went on to state that 'it is inconsistent with human dignity that a woman should use her uterus for financial profit and treat it as an incubator for someone else's child'.[22]

This, of course, is exactly how the process is described by its advocates. Surrogates have claimed that they never regarded the child as 'theirs'. The result of such a mentality, with the characterisation of surrogacy as womb-leasing, may be said to represent a mechanistic view of maternity and child-bearing, in which a mother is transformed and trivialised into a gestation machine, her integrity as a person subordinated to physical specifications: genes for fair hair and blue eyes, a pelvis suited to easy delivery. A woman becomes a factory, the unknown and uncared-for entity that will produce a child for the customer, with satisfaction guaranteed.

The objections to the use of human beings as merely compilers of body parts can be further extended if we return to the analogy considered earlier, in which surrogacy was compared with various forms of employment. It was argued that the demands made upon surrogates go far beyond those contemplated by ordinary employment. It is not unreasonable to argue that such an intrusion into a woman's privacy by regulating the intimate details of her life, combined with the notion of a service that cannot be terminated by the 'employee', are reminiscent of slavery. Certainly, the biblical models cited as examples of the historical tradition of surrogacy were both predicated upon a mistress–slave relationship of obligation. Using this analogy, surrogacy may not be merely undesirable, but actually infringe laws against slavery. Even if it falls short of breaking a law, surrogate motherhood raises once again the proposition that one person (not just her abilities, but her entire being) is being 'used' by another.

3. SOLUTIONS

If surrogacy for reward is merely deemed to be a form of employment, it ought probably to attract no greater legal regulation than any other type of work. If, however, as has been argued, it is more closely analogous either to a sort of slavery or to the sale of a bodily organ contrary to public policy, then steps ought to be taken to define the unlawful aspects of the transactions and to prevent these from continuing.

The Warnock report responded to the problems it perceived in surrogacy by proposing that the creation or operation of surrogate agencies should be rendered criminal, as should the actions of professionals or others assisting in the process. It has been suggested, however, that it is not so much the presence of an agency as its commercial nature, the inducement of money, that provides the coercive or unlawful element of the transaction. The Government's bill, referred to earlier, attempts to respond to such concerns by making criminal only the acts of those intermediaries who assist in surrogate arrangements in exchange for payment. But, this seems to miss the real issue. The most troublesome aspect of commercialisation is not the payment to the agency, but the payment to the surrogate. Under the Warnock committee's proposals and the measures in the bill, a wealthy couple or voluntary organisation would still be able to offer large sums of money to an impoverished or dependent woman, to enter into the sort of arrangement already condemned for its degrading and possibly unlawful nature. On the other hand, a helpful physician, psychologist or even commercial agency who charged a fee for assistance in screening or counselling a volunteer surrogate, would be liable for prosecution.

The Warnock committee's proposals would, however, work positively in two ways to meet the possibility of exploitation and abuse of surrogates. First, there is no doubt that the banning of commercial agencies would curtail the volume of surrogate transactions, and with it there ought to be a lower probability that things will go wrong. Secondly, the surrogacy arrangements which do continue will be hidden from public view. Presumably, if people do not hear about surrogate motherhood it will not figure among the options considered.

Are these solutions appropriate responses to perceived unlawfulness, or merely a form of hypocrisy, an 'out of sight, out of mind' approach to a serious social problem? The law would be unlikely to tolerate slavery, even if it were quietly and privately arranged. Similarly, society would frown upon kidney sales, even in small numbers. Why, then, does the Warnock committee propose such a simplistic and ineffective response to surrogacy?

C. The child

Perhaps the most compelling of all criticisms of surrogate motherhood is that it may somehow be damaging to the children involved. Again, this problem may be divided into two components: tangible harms to specific children and assaults upon our notions of childhood and the parent–child relationship in general.

1. THREATS POSED TO 'SURROGATE CHILDREN'

i. The absence of a 'normal' family
In the best of all worlds, we would wish to grant to every child opportunity to be born as the natural offspring of married parents and raised in a loving home by the same couple, comfortable, secure and self-assured.

For the child born as the result of a surrogate transaction, some of the elements of this ideal family life will be missing. The obvious departure from the normal state of affairs is the fact that the adults who raise the child will not be his biological parents. In fact, these 'social parents' need not meet any of the normal physical requirements imposed by nature on ordinary parents. There may, for example, only be one known parent, or two 'parents' of the same sex, or the adults may be otherwise obviously incapable of normal parenthood. Among the first potential clients of one American surrogacy lawyer were a seventy-year-old woman and a transsexual (each with an accompanying male partner to inseminate the surrogate).[23]

These arrangements may not be to a child's benefit. However, it has been suggested, even by such supporters of the traditional family as the Roman Catholic church, that society's model of the happy nuclear family may be no more than an 'ad-man's myth'.[24] It is estimated that 30 per cent of the children of natural parentage are not raised by the adults who conceived them.[25] A happy and caring 'surrogate family' may seem in many ways preferable to some existing forms of parentage (for example, that resulting when a man fathers a child in a brief liaison with a woman who is not at all suited to motherhood).

The motivation of couples choosing to commission a surrogate has often been criticised. Prospective parents are seen as desperate to go to any extent to ensure that they obtain 'their' child through surrogacy and some have asked whether such desperation is a good basis for parenthood.[26] Their fears may be justified, but it may also be said that many existing children could benefit from having been desperately desired by their parents, to the extent of being willing to pay £13,000 for the privilege of parenthood.

ii. Potential failure of the transactions
Given the emotionally-charged nature of surrogacy transactions, there is always the fear that something may go wrong. Again, this is a risk present to some extent in every child's life. The possibility of being born defective and rejected by parents is not peculiar to surrogacy, nor are the problems of parental custody disputes. Any child's father may die before the birth. Any mother may eschew proper pregnancy care or ingest substances that may be harmful to the fetus. The commonly discussed surrogacy 'horror stories' (What if no one wants it? What if the parents fight over it?) can all be found in everyday life. But there is a danger with surrogacy that such occurences may be more frequent and more complicated. There is also the notion, equally applicable in considering surrogacy's deviation from the 'ideal family', that an admission of existing problems ought not to be cited as justification for the encouragement of similar difficulties in future.

iii. Psychological harms
In many ways, the emotional difficulties potentially facing the child born to a surrogate are similar to those which face some adopted children. There may be a certain confusion about his identity resulting from ignorance of his background.

Conversely, if the child knows who his surrogate mother is, the confusion may stem instead from a concern as to which woman is his 'real mother'.

For the child who is a product of such as unusual arrangement, the very nature of his provenance may also create a distinct sense of unease. The mere fact of being different from ordinary children can itself be a source of difficulty and the notion of surrogacy may be hard to comprehend. There are many adults who feel a certain sense of repulsion at the suggestion that children can be the objects of commercial transactions. The fact that babies can be bought and sold (and what child could understand the subtle distinctions argued?) is likely to be even more unsettling to those who are the product of such an arrangement. 'How much did I cost? (and why not more?). How could my "real mother" have given me up for money? (or even out of generosity?) Do my parents ever wish they could get their money back?' Fear that he may be the object of a future sale may seriously threaten a child's security. However, at least in this case, parents may sensitively choose the moment at which they inform the child of the circumstances of his birth. The same opportunity is not afforded the children of the surrogate herself, who watch their mother go through her pregnancy, then see that the child is given away. Will they be next?

Some, however, are remarkably adaptable to the concept. The story is told of a surrogate mother who explained to her nine-year old daughter that the baby she was carrying would be given to another family. Matter-of-factly, the girl responded, 'All right ... but if it's a girl, let's keep it and give Jeffrey [her two-year-old brother] away!'[27]

iv. Possible legal responses

The three problems discussed above suggest that surrogate motherhood may result in harm to two categories of children. In the first group are those actually born to surrogate mothers and who may be threatened by physical or psychological hardship as a result. In the second category come children already in existence who have some connection with adults participating in a surrogacy transaction.

The harmful influence which an act or event may have upon

existing children is quite frequently cited as a legitimate reason for drafting legislation against it. One such example is the UK Abortion Act of 1967, section 1(1)(a) of which states that a pregnancy may be terminated if its continuation would involve risk of injury to the physical or mental health of existing children of the mother's family. Anti-surrogacy measures might presumably be based on this rationale alone.

How, though, ought the law to respond to the argument that there are risks that threaten children born as the result of a surrogacy arrangement?

In general, the state does not pry into the personal affairs of the family. Parents are not obliged always to do that which is in their children's best interests. Only when they reject, abuse, neglect or dispute the custody of their children will there be considered sufficient justification for the state to investigate or intervene in family arrangements. The bond between parent and child is considered the core of the family and the continued existence of the family as a strong institution is of great importance to society. There is no artificial creation of the state which is felt to be as good at child-rearing as parents.

However, when the model of the family is significantly altered, the trust society feels it can place in the family may be weakened. In many cases, it is difficult to remedy the problem of abnormally-constituted families. Attempting to prohibit the conception of children outside a normal family relationship, for example, would be pointless. We simply have to hope that the natural physical bond between mother and child will foster an atmosphere conducive to caring parentage. But when no natural physical bond exists, society may well feel justified in intervening in order to avoid the sort of harm to the child that may result if appropriate emotional bonds do not replace those ordinarily provided by nature. And if this is so, the question then becomes one of determining the proper means, if any, of such intervention.

Should the conception of 'surrogate babies' be outlawed, on the ground that such an unusual sort of provenance may have detrimental effects upon the children who result from it? It can, of course, be argued that children born of natural reproduction may, and sometimes do, run greater risks of harm, but this is not an argument in favour of encouraging surrogacy.

The unavoidable incidence of undesirable forms of natural parentage may be quite different from facilitating the creation of potential problem families when this can be avoided. Thus, there is a strong argument in favour of forbidding outside intervention, especially any sort of state-supported intervention, in performing inseminations or otherwise facilitating surrogate transactions.

It is more difficult to justify sanctions against parents who resort to surrogate motherhood, if such sanctions are to be based simply on the potential risks of harm to the resulting children. By analogy, courts have consistently refused to award damages in actions for 'wrongful life' where a child is born with a handicap that was negligently overlooked in prenatal testing.[28] Despite the negligence, despite the fact that the child's mother would have chosen to abort the child had she known of the defect, the courts have taken the view that it is better for a child to be born, albeit disabled, than not to have lived at all.

This is a sensible doctrine to apply to children who have already been born. It seems wrong to suggest that such children ought never to have existed. The argument loses some of its force, however, when considered with regard to children whose conception has yet to occur. In questioning the merits of bringing such children into existence, we do not face the problem of passing judgement that a living person would actually be better off dead. For example, we may fully appreciate the worth of the life of a handicapped child and yet still support (even applaud), the decision of known carriers of genetic defects not to have children who may be born with the same handicap. Despite such a view, it is unthinkable that we would make a law to prevent the latter, or anyone else, from conceiving, no matter how serious the potential handicap or how fragmented the family concerned. The conclusion must be, therefore, that it is inconsistent to base a law against surrogacy entirely on any potential harm to the children born through the practice.

This does not mean, however, that we are prohibited from trying to ensure that children conceived in this manner will be adequately cared for. In cases, such as adoption, where the natural, physical bonds between parent and child are absent, society feels it is justified in intervening in order to promote the formation of appropriate emotional bonds in their stead. Thus, we acknowledge the right of state agencies to screen parents wishing to adopt. Surely, it is only reasonable that we should apply the same procedure to surrogacy, at least with regard to the commissioning mother, the non-biological parent? Although it may not be appropriate to treat the father differently from any other natural father, there is no assurance that his wife or partner either can or is interested in forming a maternal relationship with the child. It would seem unusual to insist on such careful screening of adoptive parents, whilst ignoring it entirely in the case of surrogacy.

2. THREATS POSED TO OUR VIEW OF PARENTS AND CHILDREN

There is a wider proposition, going beyond specific detriments to individual children, which suggests that there is something inherent in surrogate motherhood that threatens society's basic attitudes towards childhood, the parent–child relationship and parental responsibility.

i. Constructive abandonment
One of the first surrogate mothers is said to have asked, in contemplation of the agreement to act as surrogate, whether her act was not, in essence, one of premeditated abandonment.[29] Can it ever be morally justifiable to participate in the creation of a child and of a maternal relationship for the express purpose of giving these up?

The law has developed an extensive body of parental duties and responsibilities. Chief among them is the duty of parents to care for and support their offspring throughout childhood. Neglect of this duty is a criminal offence.[30] In allowing adoption, the law acknowledges that, under circumstances thrust upon a mother, be they physical, psychological or economic, she may feel obliged to entrust the rearing of her child to others. This may not be a morally commendable action, but it is a matter of practical necessity and it also means that children will be adequately cared for. Surrogate motherhood, instead, contemplates that women first seek to initiate and then systematically to deny the responsibilities regarded as an integral part of motherhood. If the abandonment of a child constitutes a crime under existing law and the mother–child bond is at the core of our notion of the family, then it seems illogical to permit a deliberate sundering of the parental relationship in this manner.

Advocates of surrogacy have argued that the woman is bearing the child not in order to abandon it, but to give it, in what may be an act of great charity, to a couple who have a deep desire to assume responsibility for it. Thus, the child is conceived in love and given of the same love.

This proposition is open to doubt on at least two grounds. The first questions the appropriateness of the use of the words 'charity' and 'love'. Our society has consistently held that the charity and love of a parent find their expression in the exercise of parental responsibilities and duties. It is not enough to assume that someone else will love the child. Such an attitude violates the essence of the trust we put in parenthood. The surrogate mother, of course, should not be condemned too harshly for failing to perceive the serious implications of her acts; she may herself be in unfortunate straits. This, however, does not mean that the state should also refrain from considering the consequences of surrogacy.

The second ground is equally fundamental. The object of the 'gift of love' to which some refer is not a commodity, nor even a bodily organ. It is another independent life, one which we ought not to treat as largesse. A parent has no right to dispose of his child; the only real rights of parenthood are those necessary to exercise the duties arising out of the parent–child relationship.

The law has consistently held that the rights and duties of parenthood cannot be assigned to others without legal process. In the limited context of adoption, the state selects and carefully screens the transferee. When an illegitimate child is born (and all surrogate children would be so characterised because they would be born to a mother not married to their father), the mother is sole possessor of all parental rights with respect to the child, including the right to custody.[31] The only means by which she may transfer this right of custody and the duties that go with it to the child's father is by court order.[32] To make her own arrangements, including the exchange of money, would appear, as the law stands, to be a clear infringement of the law and contrary to public policy.

ii. Children as products
Among the potential consequences of an increasing availability of surrogacy is the fear that children will come to be seen as objects or commodities. This is seen in the suggestion that children can be regarded as gifts from one adult to another. It is exacerbated when the child is viewed as the product of an expensive and complicated business transaction. The screening of potential surrogate mothers to arrive at the most desirable genetic background and the most responsible prenatal nurture, must lead at least some to regard the child as a 'made to order' item of manufacture. If the 'dream child' results, this can be a very happy arrangement. However, there is an inescapable suggestion that, when effort and money are expended, value, defined by reference to the ideal, is expected.

This attitude was manifested at an American surrogacy conference, held in California in 1981, where prospective commissioning parents were overheard anxiously considering the possibility of a handicapped child: 'Will we have to take it?' The prospective surrogates responded, 'We sure don't want to be stuck with it!'[33] It seems only natural that if a child does not measure up to specifications (and no child is perfect), there will be a temptation to feel short-changed, to think in terms of fault rather than accident and to attribute most of the fault to the surrogate.

The surrogate mother, unfettered by bonds of duty and love, may well herself adopt a business-like attitude towards the pregnancy, intent on 'producing the goods' with as little trouble and effort as she can get away with. Or, she may cheat on minor terms of the agreement: 'Why not sneak a few drinks or cigarettes here and there? They'll never know!'

iii. Means and ends
A further implication of the view of children as objects is that it seems to legitimise a concept otherwise abhorrent to our way of thinking about human rights: that it is permissible to use people as means, rather than considering each as an end in himself. The law has attempted to prohibit activities which

blatantly suggest that parents are 'using' their children to serve interests other than those of the offspring themselves. For example, parents may not send their young children out to work to provide for the financial needs of the family.[34] By the same token, giving up a child for reward must be even more worthy of prohibition. It completely reduces the child to the status of a product to be used as a means to its mother's financial gain.

This is an obvious example. Less distasteful, but equally problematical from a philosophical standpoint, is the use of a child as a means by which a woman can express her generosity to a childless couple. Although one of her motives in giving away the newborn infant may be to see it raised in a good and loving home, the fact remains that the child was not conceived for its own sake, but in order that it might be the vehicle of its mother's kindness. We have in modern times abandoned the notion that children are their fathers' chattels. Today, we see the parent–child relationship as one of love and affinity that enables the protection of a younger and weaker person by those able to care for his welfare. Both parents and child, however, are persons with equal dignity and equal rights. The relationship between product and maker, product and recipient, may be perfectly smooth, even happy, but it is fundamentally a relationship of inequality.

This may appear a philosophical nicety, but in reality it goes to the root of society's aims in protecting the family. Children are individuals and the compendium of parental duties reflects one intent: that the child is a human being who should be treated in a way as to acknowledge and encourage his integrity as such. The erosion of this concept inherent in surrogate mother transactions may in many cases seem imperceptible. Individual 'surrogate children' may appear to flourish in the homes of their commissioning parents and to be treated as fully autonomous persons. What is objectionable, though difficult to isolate in specific cases, is the subtle change in society's attitudes that results when we remove the absolute duty upon parents to care for the children they bear and allow these children to be treated as objects of commerce or gifts. In doing so, we threaten both the dignity of individuals and the security of the family.

D. Arguments against surrogacy: a review

Having explored some of the objections to surrogacy raised in the Warnock committee's report, several points emerge as particularly problematical. Specifically, these are:

1. that paid surrogacy may be exploitative of the women concerned in that the amount of money offered may overcome the normal, expected refusal to submit to such an onerous invasion of their private lives;

2. that it may be against public policy to permit the transfer of money in respect of the use of the woman's body, in particular her womb;

3. that surrogacy violates the principles of maternal responsibility;

4. that it entails the use of children as means rather than regarding them as ends in themselves;

5. that it may potentially cause distress to children who are witnesses of the process.

Taken together, these points certainly appear to provide sufficient justification for imposing restrictions of at least some sort on surrogacy. Thus, it is suggested that, in general terms, the Warnock committee's negative response to surrogacy was quite appropriate. The difficulty, however, with the proposals outlined in the report is that they do not seem to meet the specific problems identified as arising in surrogacy. If we consider, for example, that, as has been suggested, the exchange of money for the use of a bodily organ is contrary to public policy, then the appropriate solution would seem to be a ban on all paid surrogacy. If we also believe that it is impermissible for a woman to conceive a child for the purpose of giving it away, this suggests that all surrogacy, paid or voluntary, should be prohibited. And, if another major area of concern is the welfare of children born to surrogate mothers, then, if the practice is to continue in any fashion, it must be regulated so as to ensure that welfare. None of these conclusions was reached by the Warnock committee.

The recommendations proposed in the report and adopted in the government's bill introduced in 1985 attack, instead, only that which is superficially distasteful about surrogate motherhood. The effect of the provisions would be to reduce the volume of surrogacy transactions but sweep the remainder out of sight, where the real problems would be beyond society's ability to respond to or to remedy.

ALTERNATIVE SOLUTIONS

A. Total prohibition

How, then, *ought* the issue of surrogacy to be settled? If we are convinced by the argument that no one should be permitted deliberately to avoid her maternal responsibilities, either for love or money, then the obvious solution is to attempt to devise a method of preventing all surrogacy transactions.

This, of course, raises tremendous practical difficulties. First, it is quite possible that couples may be sufficiently determined to have children by surrogacy that they will opt for the practice regardless of whether or not it is prohibited. Secondly, if the law were to make all surrogacy criminally unlawful, it could find itself hindered in the detection and regulation of possible harms and abuses that might result from 'underground' surrogacy. In addition, secrecy in and outside the family about the nature of a child's provenance could well undermine the stability of the families concerned and, consequently, of society.

Finally, the enforcement of laws against surrogacy, given the intimate nature of the arrangements, would be both difficult and possibly counter-productive. What sanctions could be imposed on transgressors? Fines would be unlikely to deter those intent upon paying huge sums of money for a child. If we imprison his parents for conceiving him, it will be the child who will suffer most. Similarly, his position will be jeopardised if we insist he stays with a mother who does not want him, or publicly declare him illegitimate, or refuse to allow the only family that claims his as theirs to have legal recognition as his parents. Thus, it seems that the most obvious response to the problems of surrogate motherhood may be impractical.

B. Licensing and regulation

If indeed it would not be plausible to seek to outlaw surrogacy, then thought must be given to practical methods by which surrogacy could be regulated. How could the most detrimental features of the practice be avoided? One method might be to regulate surrogate transactions by imposing a licensing scheme for agencies, requiring various forms of mandatory screening and counselling for participants.

There are serious problems with this approach. The most obvious is that government interference in, or control of, surrogacy would imply a legitimisation of the practice and perhaps act to encourage participants. If surrogacy clinics were established and licensed, it seems likely that the publicity would increase the popularity of surrogacy as a means of overcoming childlessness. If, however, it is accepted that there are serious problems inherent in surrogacy *per se*, then it is arguable that government ought to discourage rather than encourage the practice. The most serious objections to surrogacy will not be removed even if the process as a whole is subject to close scrutiny, and it would seem wrong to spend sums of public money on the licensing of an activity that has been judged to be contrary to public policy. Thus, it appears that the only legitimate form of regulation would be one which sought to eliminate aspects of surrogacy found to be particularly problematical.

C. Prohibition of commercial surrogacy

1. THE ROLE OF INTERMEDIARIES

The solution adopted by the Warnock committee and incorporated into the government's bill is to curtail surrogacy by imposing restrictions on the participation of intermediaries. No person or organisation is to initiate, take part in negotiations or compile information for use in surrogacy arrangements if such is done 'on a commercial basis' (that is, in return for payment to the intermediary).

The prohibition of commercial agencies would certainly limit the growth in the number of surrogate transactions. It would also specifically overcome the sort of abuse seen in the 'stud farms' previously described. One suspects, however, that the measure is designed more to cover up what the public finds distasteful about surrogacy (profit-hungry agencies) than to counteract any ill effects the practice may have upon its participants and on society at large. The more sensational possibilities for exploitation aside, there seems little difference, as regards most of surrogacy's problems, between a commercial agency and a volunteer one, between a transaction mediated by an agency and one conducted privately.

One of the distinctly counterproductive features of the move to curtail intermediaries recommended by the Warnock committee and found in the bill is the effective exclusion of professionals such as doctors and solicitors from surrogacy arrangements. If no person is permitted, in exchange for payment, to compile information in respect of a surrogate arrangement, then couples and prospective surrogates would not, for example, be able to consult their physicians for genetic testing. If no one may take part in the negotiations, then solicitors would not be allowed to assist in facilitating the legal adoption of children born to surrogates.

A prohibition on professional assistance adds to, rather than detracts from, the difficulties associated with surrogacy. It prevents couples from seeking advice that may either lead them to decide against surrogacy or help them to proceed in the way least prejudicial to the interests of all concerned, especially the child. Without in any way encouraging surrogacy, the availability of professional assistance could point towards an informal screening process and allow the resulting child to be properly incorporated into the family that will be caring for him.

On both sides of the Atlantic, professional bodies have already begun to prohibit their members from any form of active recruiting of surrogates.[35] This might be the most sensible way in which to regulate the participation of doctors, solicitors, psychologists and others in the surrogacy process and would be preferable to excluding them completely.

2. THE ROLE OF SURROGATES

Both the Warnock committee and the drafters of the Government's bill recognised that one of the principal problems involved in surrogacy was its commercial aspect. It is suggested, however, that they approached the problem in the wrong way. Instead of seeking to prohibit payment to those assisting in surrogacy arrangements, they should have concentrated on the prohibition of payment to surrogates themselves. Although this solution would not resolve all the fundamental objections to surrogacy, it may be the practical alternative best suited to the protection of those concerned and of society in general.

The result of such a prohibition would probably be to limit the participants in surrogacy arrangements to friends or relatives of the couple seeking a child. Few women would voluntarily bear a child for a stranger. If there were to be an additional ban on advertising, as proposed in section 3 of the bill, then strangers could not ordinarily become involved.

Such a limitation of surrogacy to voluntary arrangements may resolve beneficially a number of the problems associated with surrogacy. First, volunteers would be much less likely to be victims of financial coercion. Equally, they would be unlikely to exploit the couples involved. It is of course arguable that the emotional pressure exerted by a relative or friend could be considerable. However, emotional pressure to perform voluntarily a lawful act is not the sort of duress that is sufficiently severe as to involve sanctions of law.

Secondly, if we refer back to the criteria for organ donations, voluntary womb-leasing ought to fit within the 'approved' category, in that it is the sort of disposition that was thought to be permissible if offered as a donation, but probably contrary to public policy if done in exchange for money. Paid surrogacy, of course, would have been against public policy, according to this test.

A third issue was the disruption of the marriage of the commissioning couple by the surrogate. There is no doubt that the presence of a friend or relative as a 'third party' to the marriage may present a considerable amount of tension. Morally, however, it may be less problematical than a similar intrusion by a stranger. If ties of blood or affection bind the commissioning parents and surrogate, they suggest that the second woman already has a link with the marriage. If anyone could be deemed appropriate as a substitute for the wife, then perhaps it is someone closely related or connected to her and to the family.

The final and perhaps most serious difficulty with surrogacy was the effect of the process upon the children concerned and upon our notions of childhood. At an individual level, the insistence that surrogate transactions be unpaid might well reduce the likelihood of the agreement dissolving into a dispute detrimental to the child. The involvement of friends would result in an arrangement where participants would be inclined to understand and care about each others' interests in the process. An additional benefit is a sort of built-in screening mechanism. A woman who is acting out of love rather than money and who deals directly with the commissioning father is much more likely to ask herself whether or not he is a suitable parent and similarly to consider the prospective mother.

It has been argued, of course, that it is not fair to ask a woman to go through the hardship of a surrogate pregnancy without compensating her for the pain, inconvenience and time. Surely, the better question is whether it is fair to *ask* a woman to undergo a pregnancy for someone else *at all*, and the answer is clearly 'no'. Only if a friend, out of love or compassion, *offers* herself in such a way can the offer be tolerated as a gift of self. The surest way to limit surrogacy to the cases most likely to proceed smoothly is to require an exceptional altruism in the surrogate mother.

However, by allowing even voluntary surrogacy, it is hard to avoid the allegations that surrogacy is equivalent to constructive abandonment and entails the use of a child as the means to an end. The elimination of paid surrogacy would, of course, improve the situation somewhat. The absence of a formal contract and exchange of 'goods' for money would eliminate some of the factors leading to a child-as-product mentality. Although problems could arise either as the result of over-solicitous interference from a surrogate who was a close relative or friend, or confusion for the child as to which woman was his real mother, children might still find it easier to comprehend the idea of 'auntie helping mummy' than of a business transaction between strangers. And it is arguable that a woman who knows the family well into which her child will be adopted, or is herself a member of that family, is committing a less reprehensible act than one who gives her infant to strangers. Nevertheless, the basic philosophical objections remain and nothing short of total prohibition, dismissed as impractical, could remove them. The continuing existence of such problems must serve as a reminder that the scheme proposed here is simply a way in which some forms of surrogacy may be tolerated and not an endorsement of a process which remains fundamentally at odds with public policy.

PRACTICAL RECOMMENDATIONS

A. To prohibit commercial surrogacy

The prohibition of payment for surrogacy could be best accomplished by a statutory provision, similar to that in section 57 of the English Adoption Act (1976), which prohibits all transfers of payment in respect of the adoption of a child. It is, of course, possible that clandestine payments may be made. The chief function, however, of such a provision would be to inhibit most people from entering into the arrangement in the first place. And, if they chose to break the law, the consequences would not be as severe as would be the case if surrogacy in any form were prohibited by law. The illegality would refer only to the financial transaction and not to the very conception of the child. Enforcement could take the form of a fine levied on all parties, commensurate, in the case of the surrogate, with the amount received from the couple. Given that the transaction would be illegal, no restitution order would be granted in favour of the couple. Neither the imprisonment of the parents nor the denial to them of the custody of the child in punishment for their acts would be appropriate sanctions.

B. To deal with intermediaries

It is further suggested that the reasons of policy which may propose that a certain amount of mercy be granted to the commissioning parents and surrogate mother do not necessarily extend to any participating intermediaries. While professional counselling and medical or legal advice ought not to be discouraged, there is a case for recommending strong sanctions against professionals, individuals or agencies who actively recruit surrogates and facilitate arrangements by, for example, performing artificial insemination. To this end, a provision could be introduced prohibiting the involvement of anyone, on a commercial or non-profit basis, in the recruitment of women to act as surrogates. As an increased safeguard, the provisions of section 3 of the Surrogacy Arrangements Bill, placing a ban on advertising, could also be incorporated into the legislation.

C. To care for resulting children

If surrogacy is to occur, then, even if it is made totally or partially illegal, there is still a responsibility upon the state to ensure that any resulting children are adequately cared for. The facilitation of such care need not imply a condonation of the surrogacy arrangement itself, but could deal with the children as 'victims' of what might be an unlawful activity. In the unhappy event that the parties contest the custody of the child, the case ought to be considered as would any other custody dispute. The parties will have to come to court and have all the facts (including the circumstances of the conception and birth) weighed by the judge. The final determination will be based primarily upon what are thought to be the child's best interests.

In 'ordinary' uncontested surrogacy cases, certain changes in the law might facilitate the smoothest possible incorporation of the child into the family that is to raise him.

The law gives all rights over an illegitimate child to its mother. If the surrogate is unmarried, the child will be illegitimate. If married, the child will be presumed to be the offspring of that marriage.[36] If the parties concerned agree, this situation can be altered. A court order of affiliation can result in formal acknowledgement of the paternity of the commissioning father.[37] He can then seek custody of the child and, in some cases, will be permitted to adopt it. The process is lengthy and cumbersome and there is some uncertainty as to its successful outcome. It was certainly not designed with surrogacy in mind. In addition, there have been proposals made regarding AID that suggest that the husband of a woman who bears a child through that method of fertilisation will be irrebuttably presumed to be the child's father. This would deny to the commissioning (and biological) fathers of many surrogate children the chance even to initiate affiliation and custody proceedings.

It is recommended that a simpler procedure be adopted to deal with all cases in which a single mother wishes to give up her child to its father. Once the mother (surrogate) has made clear her intentions by making her child available for adoption, the father who desires custody should be presumed to be the person best suited to care for the child, subject to contrary evidence. Both he and his partner, if any, should be subject to some official screening process in order to ensure that they meet minimum standards of acceptability as parents. A licensed adoption agency is probably the best body to conduct such investigations. If the father is successful, adoption, and not mere custody, as is often the current practice, ought to be recommended.

Conclusion

The scheme proposed is one which attempts to set a framework for what the Warnock committee calls the 'minimum requirements for a tolerable society'.[38] Surrogate motherhood poses a difficult challenge for society and the law. Popular feeling demands that the legislature respond quickly, but such response cannot merely reflect popular feeling. The arguments against imposing restrictions on surrogacy rely on respect for liberty and autonomy, while opponents suggest that surrogacy represents a threat to human dignity that can only make us less free, less autonomous. Achieving a balance is particularly difficult when it is almost impossible to predict in advance either the full nature and extent of the challenge posed by surrogacy, or all the ramifications of any proposed solutions.

What, then, should be the next step for the government? The Warnock committee's report has set the scene by outlining in brief some of the problems posed by surrogacy. The government's bill represents a tentative step towards resolving some of them. What is needed at this point is a more comprehensive legislative response, one which takes seriously the suggestion that sentiment need not be ignored but that argument must prevail; a response that provides a reasoned analysis of the problems and a careful and thoughtful solution which will work in practice.

Notes and references

1 Genesis 1:28

2 K Bird. Surrogate motherhood: hers? yours? ours? California Lawyer, 21, February 1982.

3 C Goldfarb. Two mothers, one baby, no law. Human Rights, 11, 1983, 26.

4 The Times, 25 April 1984, page 11.

5 Genesis 16:1 tells the story of Abram, Sarai and Hagar; Genesis 30:1 that of Jacob, Rachel and Bilhah.

6 In re a baby. Times Law Report, 15 January 1985.

7 Peter Bruinvels, (C) Leicester E, quoted in The Times, 5 January 1985.

8 Quoted in: W Wadlington. Artificial conception: the challenge for family law. Va Law Review, 69, 1983, 6.

9 Department of Health and Social Security. Report of the Committee of Inquiry into Human Fertilisation and Embryology. Cmnd 9314 (Chairman: Dame Mary Warnock) London, HMSO, 1984, paragraph 8.18.

10 See 9 above, paragraph 8.17.

11 See 9 above, paragraph 8.10.

12 See 9 above, paragraphs 11.13–11.18.

13 See 9 above, Foreword.

14 See 9 above, paragraph 8.10.

15 See 9 above, paragraph 4.10.

16 See 9 above, paragraph 8.10.

17 P Coleman. Surrogate motherhood: analysis of the problem and suggestions for solutions. Tennessee Law Review, 1982, 81.

18 P Parker. Motivation of surrogate mothers: initial findings. American Journal of Psychiatry, 140, 1983, 117.
19 See, for example, A Hutchinson. Surrogate motherhood: why it should be permitted. Toronto Globe and Mail, 10 July 1985.
20 See, for example, the statement of John Patten, Parliamentary Secretary for Health, in which he says, 'I have already strongly condemned the abhorrent practice of offering human tissue [ie kidneys] for profit ... Ministers regard transplantation of an organ ordained for payment as improper and undesirable'. 10 June 1985.
21 *Perlmutter v Beth David Hospital*, 123 NE (2d) 792 (1954).
22 See 9 above, paragraph 8.10.
23 N P Keane and D L Breo. The surrogate mother. New York, Everest House, 1981.
24 Social Welfare Commission of the Catholic Bishops' Conference (England and Wales). Human fertilisation – choices for the future. March 1983.
25 J Robertson. Procreative liberty and the control of conception, pregnancy and childbirth. Va Law Review, 69, 1983, 419.
26 For example, Senator Connie Binsfield (Michigan), in a letter dated 16 March 1983, addressed to fellow Senators regarding proposed surrogacy legislation in that state.
27 Quoted in: H Krimmel. The case against surrogate parenting. Hastings Center Report, October 1983, 35.
28 For example, *McKay v Essex Area Health Authority* [1982] 2 All ER 771.
29 Quoted in Bird (see 2 above) at page 25.
30 Parliament. Children and Young Persons Act, 1933. London, HMSO, 1933, section 1.
31 Parliament. Childrens Act, 1975. London, HMSO, 1975, section 85(7).
32 Parliament. Guardianship of Minors Act, 1971. London, HMSO, 1971, section 9.
33 See 27 above, at page 37.
34 Parliament. Employment of Childrens Act, 1973. London, HMSO, 1973, section 9.

35 For example, the American College of Obstetricians and Gynecologists' statement of policy: Ethical issues in surrogate motherhood, May 1983; British Medical Association, Interim report on human in vitro fertilisation approved. British Medical Journal, 286, 1983, pages 1590–1591.

36 Parliament. Affiliation Proceedings Act, 1957. London, HMSO, 1957.

37 Parliament. Family Law Report Act, 1969. London, HMSO, 1969, section 27.

38 See 9 above, Foreword.

THE JEWISH CONTRIBUTION TO MEDICAL ETHICS

Sir Immanuel Jakobovits

As an introduction to the subject of the Jewish contribution to medical ethics, let me first point out a somewhat strange anomaly. Of all the disciplines of science and human thought, it is doubtless medicine with which Judaism, right from its very origins, has had the closest affinity, going back to the very roots of our biblical tradition.

In the Bible itself, in the Hebrew Bible, we find a good many references basic to the very foundations of medical ethics. There is the reverence for the supreme value and dignity of human life, created as man is in the image of God. The very start of the Genesis story insists on the inviolability of human life. There is the emphasis on the preservation of life and health as a religious precept, being not merely something which is, as it were, optional, but which is religiously required of us. It is in the pursuit of our duty towards our Creator that we are commanded to ensure that life and limb and health are protected from any harm. In addition there are many detailed regulations, including the dignity to be extended even to the dead, even to a capital criminal, someone who has been executed – because he too was created in the image of God and, therefore, must not be exposed to any undue humiliation or indignity, which accounts to this day for our rather restrictive attitude towards autopsies and post mortems.

So the foundations for Jewish medical ethics were laid in the Bible. It was also first in laying down a fairly advanced system of what we might call social medicine or preventive medicine, public sanitation regulations, such as the treatment of lepers, the attitude to cleanliness as being next to holiness, and a rigid code of sexual morality and hygiene. Later on, in the next great phase of the development of Jewish thought, in the Talmud – the composition of which covers some 800 years from roughly the third century before the common era, until the fifth century of the common era – we have already a great many precise definitions on medical ethics, instructions and regulations, that cover such details as, for instance, the administration of contraceptives and the attitude to therapeutic abortion. There are references in the Talmud which deal with doctor-patient relationships, with malpractice claims for compensation for injuries caused by negligence and numerous other items that constitute the wherewithall of what we nowadays term medical ethics.

This Talmudic heritage – which runs into many tomes, vast volumes comprising these 800 years of academic discussions in the academies of learning in ancient Palestine and Babylonia, the main centres of Jewish creative learning – was then further developed into the great codes of Jewish law, which all make extensive reference to items of medical-ethical interest, culminating in that of Maimonides, a great and outstanding physician mentioned in every textbook on the history of medicine. He was not only a distinguished physician but also the leading authority on Jewish law in the Middle Ages. His monumental work was followed by a further code, the final codification of Jewish law, which goes back to the sixteenth century, and by numerous commentaries, all of them replete with references to medical ethics. That was finally further evolved and augmented to the present day in what are called the rabbinic responsa, that is, questions submitted to rabbinic judgement, to leading rabbinical sages, whose replies given, usually in writing, are collected in major works, again multi-volume tomes. These are being published by the hundreds, up to this day, notably in Israel and in the United States as well as sometimes in this country and elsewhere. All these rulings, given by leading rabbinical scholars in response to modern queries submitted to their judgement, gradually establish new norms to become part of the corpus of Jewish law, binding on future generations.

Jewish medical ethics was also promoted by the very close partnership between the rabbinical and the medical professions for long periods in our history. This partnership in the Middle Ages, for instance, was so intense that it has been estimated that over half of all the best known medieval Jewish thinkers – rabbies, grammarians, philosophers, poets – were physicians by occupation, men such as Maimonides and countless others. Indeed, this tradition of a special propensity towards medicine no doubt accounts for the prominent role of Jews in the history of medicine, especially in modern times; to such an extent, that out of all the Nobel Prize winners in medicine, no fewer than 20 per cent are Jews, which is 40 times the ratio of Jews to the world's population.

In view of this, it is surprising that Jewish medical ethics as a distinct and academically recognised discipline has not come into existence until very recent times. As a matter of fact, I believe that my doctoral thesis submitted to London University in the middle fifties under the title of 'Jewish Medical Ethics', a comparative study of the attitude of religion to medicine with special reference to Judaism and later condensed in a book under the same title, was the first time that the term had ever been used. It was a generally quite unknown subject, and if you wanted to know Jewish attitudes towards any widely debated modern subjects – such as abortion, contraception or sterilisation – you would have to be fairly well-versed in Biblical and Talmudic studies to find access to all the intricate works in which these attitudes are embedded. Until recent times, nothing was available in modern form to medical students or doctors, or the enlightened public, which would provide some guidance on what Judaism had to say on these subjects.

I am glad to say that literature on the subject is now proliferating and there is quite an impressive library of works on Jewish medical ethics, largely in English, partly in Hebrew. We have several institutes, again notably in Israel, exclusively dedicated to research in, and the teaching of, Jewish medical ethics. I have recently opened the first Centre for Jewish Medical Ethics at Ben Gurion University in Beer Sheva in Israel, which I am proud to say bears my name.

These are some of the historical parameters, including the anomalies, within which the discipline of Jewish medical ethics has developed. It is now seking to assert its role in the public debate on the numerous moral issues that exercise us in the face of the spectacular advances of modern medicine. These advances raise profound moral problems that were undreamt of only a few decades ago; nevertheless, in order to find Jewish answers we will have to search for and discover precedents and principles enshrined in earlier layers of our literature.

In order to illustrate how Jewish medical ethics goes to work, utilising these earlier sources to deal with more up-to-date problems, I will concentrate on its conclusions that differ from the commonly accepted norms of medical ethics. If we merely confirm what everyone else has to say, we do not have to say it, or at least I do not have to deal with it. I want to indicate the distinctive marks of Jewish medical ethics and the divergence between Judaism and other traditions, rather than the convergence.

First, a straightforward biblical illustration. It is not often that we can fall directly on a biblical precedent. My example deals with the highly up-to-date contemporary question of whether to inform or not to inform. If you diagnose a fatal illness, should the patient be told, be informed, or can you under certain circumstances suppress the truth, or even if necessary, subvert the truth and tell a lie if he asks you straight out 'do I or don't I have cancer?' For this, we have a direct and immediate biblical precedent in the Second Book of Kings. A certain Syrian king, Ben Hadad, was dangerously ill and wanted to know his prognosis. He sent a messenger by the name of Hazaal to the land of Israel in order to consult the prophet of Israel, Elisha, to learn by divine oracle, by divine inspiration, what the outcome of his illness was likely to be. The prophet of God said to Hazaal: 'Go back to the King and inform him that he will surely live' following this affliction which he suffered; and then the prophet added: 'albeit I know that he will surely die.' There could be no more dramatic illustration of a divinely sanctioned instruction given to conceal or even falsify the truth, to hide it from the patient. On the basis of that passage, later rabbinic rulings have determined that where there is the slightest fear that, by divulging the truth, you might cause a physical or mental or psychological setback to the patient, where you may compromise the welfare of the patient, which is the first and primary consideration, then you should, if necessary, tell a downright lie, instead of allowing him to know that he is doomed according to the medical diagnosis.

This is a specifically Jewish attitude, which became cardinal to our whole attitude towards doctor patient relationships. In my experience of living on both sides of the Atlantic, doctors in America, even more than in this country, commonly would prefer to tell the truth to the patient, occasionally quite brutally, because they feel they cannot go wrong by doing so. Should the patient die in due course from a fatal disease diagnosed and communicated by the doctor, then of course the doctor is a good doctor because he made the right diagnosis. If the patient somehow survives, then the doctor is an even greater doctor because he performed a miracle. Here, it is the easiest solution for a doctor to share the confidence of his findings with the patient and to so advise him. This solution also takes account of the fact that a patient may seek notice, as it were, of impending death to prepare himself, whether spiritually by confession or, in the temporal sense, by writing his will and so on.

The Jewish attitude is that the welfare of the patient takes precedence over all other considerations, and we would gladly renounce even the opportunity for confession, which is precious to us, or any other preparation for death, if the alternative is to sap his confidence in recovery and cause him some traumatic experience which adds further ordeals of suffering to the anguish that he already experiences through his illness. This is a simple classic illustration of how the Jews go back directly to a biblical precedent to solve problems which occur in the everyday practice of medicine today.

My second illustration is not so quite straightforward, and not quite so immediate in its relationship to Jewish sources. Nevertheless, it is of direct consequence to a whole host of modern moral problems encountered in the routine administration of medicine. I refer to euthanasia in any shape or form, either the direct administration of a killing agent to a patient in distress or, by extension, the shutting-off of life support systems or any other action calculated to induce death. The whole rubric of subjects is based again on a fundamental principle, which governs the eventual solution of what may often be highly complex situations.

When the Jewish tradition speaks of the sanctity of life, as it is glibly called, it resists using abstractions or generalisations. Rather it seeks to find a more specific legal definition of something which otherwise is vague, undefined and does not lend itself to direct and immediate application in practical life. Hence, the very phrase 'sanctity of life' is an un-Jewish expression. There is no Hebrew parallel for it, neither in the Bible or the Talmud. It is something that is alien to the Jewish way of thinking.

Jews define the value, the worth of life, as being infinite. The emphasis is on the infinity of the value of every innocent human life. Infinity by definition is indivisible, however often you divide infinity, every fraction of infinity remains infinite. A millionth of infinity still is infinite. Hence, if seventy years of life are of infinite value, it follows that every part of that seventy years – thirty-five years, one year, one day, one hour, a split second – has the same infinite value. Every fraction of life is worth as much as the totality of life.

Why do Jews insist on this particular definition of the value of life? It may of course be perfectly acceptable according to the rules of mathematics or of logic, but what are the moral underpinnings of this formulation of the preciousness of the worth of human life? There is a very basic reasoning and perhaps none can sense it more acutely than Jews, who have been exposed as a people to the denial of this principle.

Let us say that a patient has one more hour to live, and that one hour, possibly accompanied by a great deal of physical suffering, being practically worthless, can be shortened. If we can hasten the demise of this patient by robbing him of one practically worthless hour, it would then follow that another patient who has not one more hour, but two, has twice that infinitesimal value; consequently, others who can expect another three months, another six months, another year, another five years, or another 10 years, would correspondingly increase in value. The result would be that no two human beings would have identical value, that we would all only have a relative value, relative either to our expectancy of life, or relative to our state of health, or relative to our contribution to society, or to any other arbitrary criterion. This leads directly and inescapably to the Nazi doctrine of grading human beings, whereby some are more important than others. Some are worth preserving at all costs, like the Teutonic race, and others are inferior races, like Jews and Gypsies who can be shoved into the ovens by the millions because they are worthless.

Therefore, if we let go on this one patient who still has one more hour to live and were to say that his hour is practically worthless, then we would drag down with him from the infinitely high pedestal on which every human being stands all other human beings, because life would no longer have an absolute value but only a relative value, relative to any of the criteria I have mentioned. Since this is unacceptable, we can never accept the deliberate termination of any innocent human life – by the administration of an overdose of lethal drugs, or injection of air into veins, or whatever. Jews are profoundly concerned to avoid and reduce human pain and human suffering, to the extent that we would gladly sacrifice many of our most precious religious observances, the Sabbath and the Day of Atonement and so on, in order to do so. The one thing that we cannot do is purchase relief from suffering at the cost of life itself – to kill a patient in order to relieve him from suffering. Thus, positive euthanasia, any action calculated to induce death, would be regarded in Jewish law as first degree murder, a direct act of killing, including any action, such as switching off a machine, intended to shorten life or hasten death.

What the masters of Jewish law at the present time are prepared to consider – and it is still a moot question currently under debate – is a possible permission, under very carefully defined circumstances, to withdraw artificial means to prolong a lingering life. Let us say you had a cancer patient who, on top of his cancer, contracts a serious infection, pneumonia, which could be suppressed by the administration of drugs, of antibiotics; and assume that you are dealing with the terminal stage of life. In that case Jewish law might not require the physician to apply these artificial means of suppressing the infection, but allow nature to take its course without artificially prolonging the dying agony. In other words, the suspension of intervention to delay death may be sanctioned, according to some of our leading authorities. But each case would have to be very carefully and responsibly examined on the strength of the best available competent medical opinion and, in the case of a patient who wishes to be guided by Jewish teachings, of equally competent rabbinic or moral opinion, concerning what is, after all, a capital verdict.

I have explained that infinity cannot be divided – every fraction of life remains infinite in value. Equally, infinity cannot be multiplied. A thousand times infinity, or a million times infinity, is no more than infinity. Jews would therefore never sanction the deliberate sacrifice of one human being, even if we knew for certain that by this sacrifice we could save a million others. For the million others are worth no more or no less than the one to be sacrificed.

Consequently, medical experiment on humans, involving life hazards, could never be sanctioned, despite the certainty of its outcome. It could only be contemplated if the first beneficiary of an experimental treatment would be the patient himself. In other words, in a desperate gamble to save a life, when no known cure is available, by all means apply an experimental cure in the hope that the life of this person, this subject on whom you carry out the experiment, may be saved. If it is saved, then of course you can apply the lessons learnt to a million others later on.

However, we can no more volunteer our own lives than we can sacrifice anybody else's life. We are only custodians of our lives, trustees not owners. Therefore the patient himself has no more right to dispose of his life, to surrender his life, or to give instructions that it shall be surrendered, than he has of anyone else's life. Volunteering for possibly fatal experiments does not lessen the moral opposition that would be encountered from a Jewish point of view.

Now to move from the termination of life, the terminal stage of life, to the inception of life. I suppose these days this raises even more highly topical arguments, controversy and public debate. What with the latest discussions on the Warnock committee report relating to *in vitro* fertilisation, artificial insemination, the cloning of human beings, genetic engineering, experiments on embryos, surrogate mothers, there are a whole host of problems undreamt of just a few years ago. These problems are now commonplace and are likely to be greatly accentuated by the continuing enormous strides being made by medical research on a scale that leaves us breathless and makes it very hard for ethicists or moralists to keep abreast with the latest advances. Again I can only spell out one or two basic principles.

The fundamental definition of life being infinite in value ceases at the moment of death as we define it – that is, the cessation of all spontaneous life functions, certainly of breathing and pulsation; not clinical death but biological death. In Jewish law, this infinite value starts from the moment of birth. In fact, the moment was very precisely defined in our literature 2000 years ago, in the early part of the Talmud, as the moment either the head or greater part of the body of the child emerges from the birth canal. From that moment, the child has the same value as any other existing human being and cannot be destroyed even to save the life of the mother – or for that matter of anyone else. However, before that moment, while we attach a very precious value to the unborn child and would only under the most exceptional circumstances be entitled to terminate a pregnancy, it is nevertheless regarded as a potential human being only, and therefore, in the event for instance of any mortal conflict between mother and child before birth, where a continued pregnancy might cause a risk of life to the mother, we would have no hesitation, no qualms of any kind, not only in sanctioning the destruction of her unborn child in order to save the mother, but in requiring it, making it mandatory to destroy this unborn life in order to save the existing life of the mother.

Accordingly, we have no hesitation in considering therapeutic abortions where indicated for grave medical reasons. I will not go into the grey areas where the threat is not to the mother's life, but to her health, or where the threat is not to the mother at all but to the child being born with grave abnormalities, such as when the mother had contracted german measles or taken drugs like thalidomide. These are areas on which there is still a great deal of debate going on in Jewish literature. But in principle we adopt a lenient attitude towards abortion since there is a medically established risk to the mother that would ensue from not intervening and allowing the pregnancy to continue.

It follows that in a great many instances we would draw a clear line of demarcation between the infinite preciousness of the life of the mother or of any other human being, and that attaching to an embryo or a fetus until the moment of birth. This, of course, is not to say we would lightly allow the destruction of a germinating life, long before it is ready for delivery and before it is indeed medically called viable, capable of living on its own. Quite exceptional circumstances apart, we would strongly object to any wastage of the potential of life. We therefore take a very severe view against allowing the male semen or the female egg, the ovum, to be deliberately destroyed, or used for anything except the sole purpose of procreation, for the sake of which we were endowed with our reproductive faculties, literally as partners with God in the generation of human life.

What we seek under the circumstances, however, is to preserve the identity of every human being, with the certain knowledge, or the capacity of finding out for certain, as to who are the father and the mother of a child, and therefore by extension the immediate blood-relations. We have to know this not just for operating the laws of incest – in order to establish who is a brother, who is a sister, who is an uncle, who is a niece – but deem it the birthright of every human being we bring into the world, so that we do not for instance, deliberately breed orphans. Embryos or semen or fertilised eggs can now be frozen and used years later, even when the donor, the husband, is long dead, and when it will suit the mother better to have a child. Such a notion is utterly repugnant to us. It is sad enough when, in the course of events, children happen to be orphaned, but deliberately to deprive a child of an identifiable father and mother is something that undermines the whole concept of the preciousness and sanctity of the generation of life, according to our Jewish insight.

Altogether, we are utterly opposed to any third-party intrusion into the exclusiveness of a marriage, which of course, excludes artificial insemination by donor (AID). There is an additional hazard in this practice. Not only does the child not know its identity, but society itself is defrauded. The Warnock report recommended that a child conceived by AID should be registered on a birth certificate as the legitimate child of the barren husband of the mother, a husband who never in fact could have a child, who was infertile; yet he should be registered as the father of the child. This means, that if some five per cent of all marriages are eligible for AID because of their infertility, then we conceal not only the truth of the paternity of this five per cent, misrepresenting who their fathers are, but make uncertain the paternity of the other 95 per cent, because once it became legal to issue fraudulent birth certificates the majority would be thrown into doubt; we would never know whether a birth certificate is truthful or not. Therefore Jews are utterly opposed to allowing this deception of society, as well as of the child concerned, to be officially sanctioned.

I might illustrate my point by referring to a case from Los Angeles recently reported in the *Sunday Express*. A middle-aged man was about to marry a twenty-year-old bride. The father of the bride felt that it was only right before the marriage was solemnised to inform his son-in-law-to-be that this bride of his, his daughter, was born by artificial insemination. The groom immediately became rather agitated, asked where it was done and so on, and discovered the hospital in which the insemination took place. He also discovered that he was the donor – the father of his bride-to-be. He was the biological father, what we would regard in Jewish law as the legal father, of this women together with 400 other children whom he had generated, whom he had sired, twenty years earlier when he was a medical student and made his semen available at that particular hospital. This is not a freak case; it is an event that can happen. But even if it could not happen, the deception that is involved here, as well as the intrusion into the exclusiveness of the marital bond, is something that horrifies Jews. We would therefore strongly object to such practices as part of our contribution to the public debate on this very sacred area of the generation of human life.

The Jews were once charged to be moral pioneers, to turn spiritual engineering into our national purpose. We were in fact a very lonely people, living in a pagan society which shared none of our convictions. Nevertheless we upheld, and later spread, notions utterly alien to the ancient world – notions like the brotherhood of man, social justice, the equality of human life, all of which were completely unknown in antiquity. We preserved our heritage not only in the face of loneliness, but of national suffering and indeed of martyrdom, and eventually helped to give birth to other great monotheistic faiths, Christianity 2000 years ago and Islam 600 years later, which now bring the inspiration of the moral order and spiritual values into hundred of millions of homes all over the world. If we have persevered in the face of all these tribulations and the enormous suffering we have endured, and have seen the fulfilment of our national dream to resurrect our collective identity, go back to our land, the land of our origin, the land of the prophets, the land whence all these teachings spread into the world, then it can only be for the ultimate purpose of resuming this historic assignment, making our contribution, along with the contribution of every other people, towards the betterment of the human condition, and the eventual establishment of a human society in which we are all brothers by virtue of having a common Father, and in which every human being will not only be created in the image of God but will live in His image.

UNEMPLOYMENT AND HEALTH

Stephen Farrow

Epidemiology and community medicine offer two distinct approaches to studying the problem of unemployment and health. Epidemiology is mainly concerned with the causes of disease and tries to disentangle the absolute and relative risks following exposure to particular environmental factors. Community medicine is the professional discipline which grew out of the old public health and is involved in the assessment of need, and the provision and management of health services. It is also the discipline which tackles the question of health policy in relation to disease prevention. This paper seeks to analyse the relationship between unemployment and ill health and discusses the factors which should be considered in making a judgement about cause and effect. Two of the standard epidemiological approaches to problem solving have been described as footleather and armchair epidemiology. In general the footleather approach requires the collection of original information. The armchair approach is usually to search the literature and to study data secondhand. This analysis is very much in the armchair tradition but has required a certain movement between libraries in order to cover the very wide range of disciplines involved. These include sociology, economics, econometrics, psychology, social psychology and health.

My starting point is the assertion that there is an association between unemployment and ill health and this paper considers some of the more recent evidence. Platt and Kreitman described the relationship between unemployment and para-suicide between 1967 and 1983.[1] Patients referred to their specialist unit who were diagnosed as para-suicide, were

Figure 1 Association in time

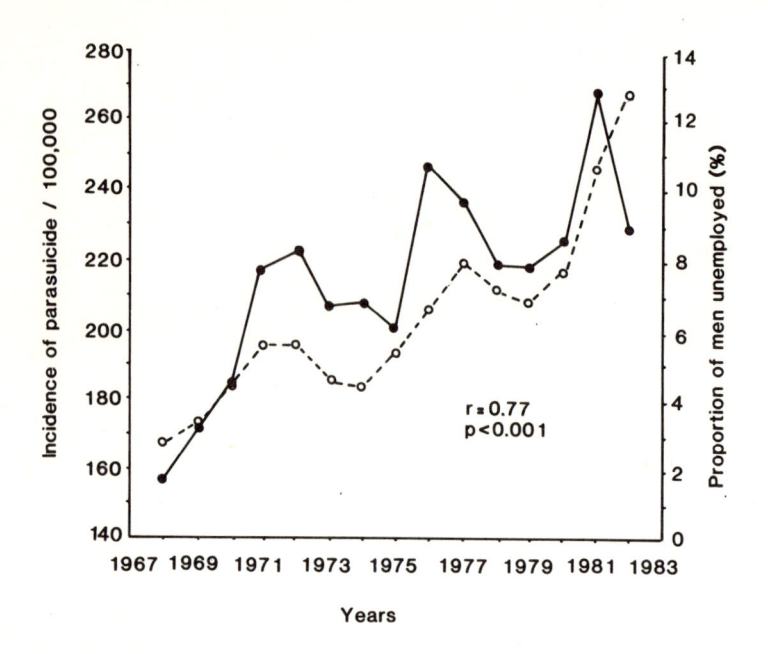

Figure: Unemployment (o---o) and incidence of parasuicide (●——●) in men in Edinburgh (1968-82). r = 0.77, p < 0.001.

from Platt & Kreitman 1984

counted, and registrations in all of the unemployment offices in Edinburgh were recorded over the same time period. Figure 1 shows the relationship in time and appears to suggest an association. The correlation coefficient was 0.77. Figure 2 from the same study shows the association in terms of place. Unemployment and para-suicides were analysed by home address in 31 electoral divisions. The correlation coefficient was 0.95, suggesting that the association was not likely to have occurred by chance.

A study from OPCS described the mortality of 500,000 people, a one per cent sample of the 1971 census. Employment status was categorised as employed, unemployed (sick), unemployed (seeking work), retired, permanently sick, student

Figure 2 Association in place

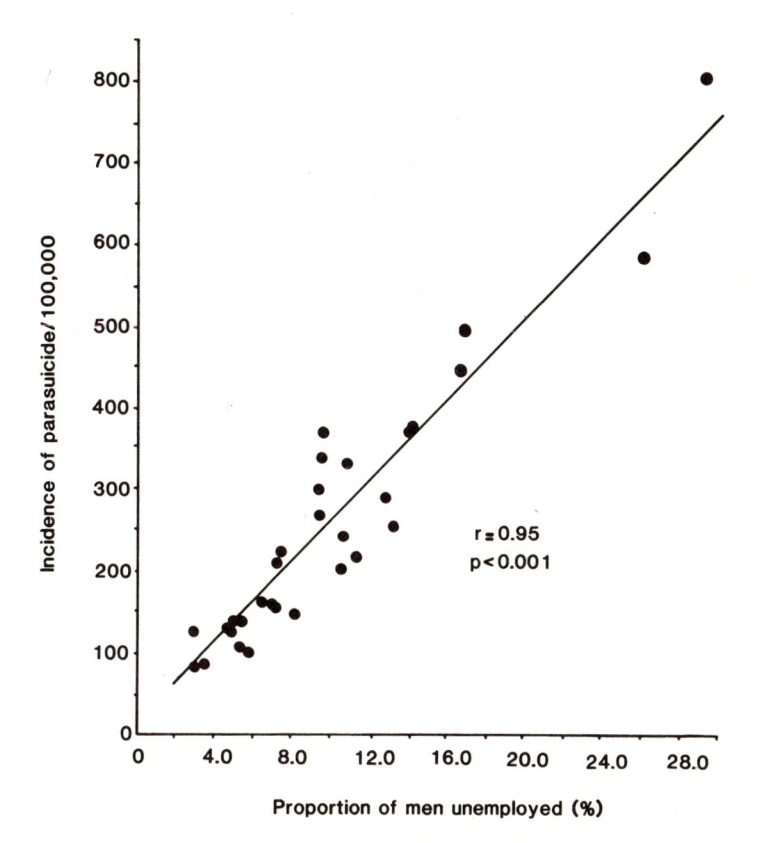

[Scatter plot: Incidence of parasuicide/100,000 vs Proportion of men unemployed (%). r = 0.95, p < 0.001]

Relation between male unemployment (1981 Census) and parasuicide in men across 31 regional electoral divisions in Edinburgh 1980-2

from Platt & Kreitman 1984

or other. Information about death and cancer registration was obtained during the next five[2] and ten years.[3] This longitudinal study provides us with moderately good evidence of an association between employment status and subsequent death. Amongst the inactive, those permanently sick had a standardised mortality ratio (SMR) of 400. On the active side, those

Figure 3 Mortality of males age 15–64 by economic position

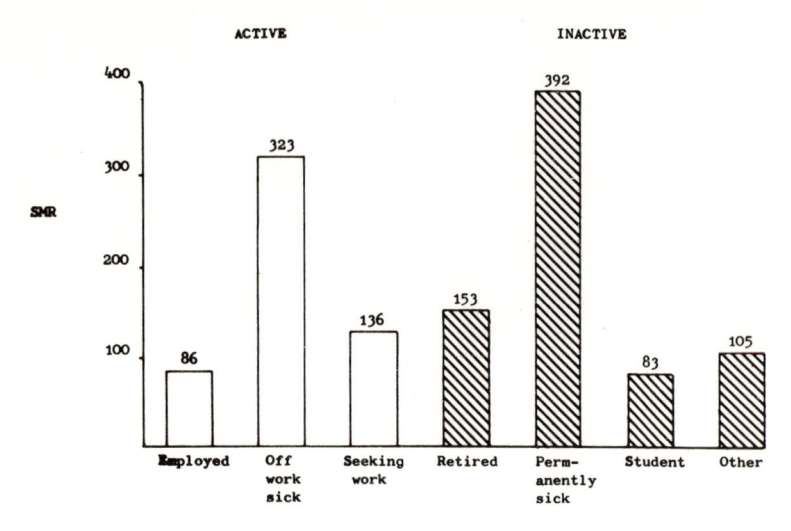

ACTIVE   INACTIVE

SMR

Employed 86
Off work sick 323
Seeking work 136
Retired 153
Permanently sick 392
Student 83
Other 105

From Fox and Goldblatt 1982

unemployed but seeking work had an SMR of 136 compared with those employed of 86 (Figure 3). Although the average SMR was 136 it does appear that people in the 35–44 age range had a slightly higher risk of dying than younger or older people. Although I have presented only two recent studies on the association between unemployment and ill health there is a great deal of evidence which has been reviewed elsewhere.[4] Perhaps the more important question is: 'Does unemployment *cause* ill health?'

The problem of causality is of concern to epidemiologists as well as to others in the field of law and ethics. There are several criteria that need to be applied when judging whether an association is causal. These include the strength of the association, biological gradient, consistency, relationship in time, plausibility and the quality of the experimental evidence.

Strength of association

The study by Doll and Hill[5] of the smoking habits of doctors 30 years ago showed not just that smoking was associated with lung cancer but that the relative risk of dying of lung cancer if you smoked was of the order of 10 times. This compared with the relative risk of 2 of dying of coronary heart disease amongst smokers. In the case of unemployment and health the relative risk appears to be 1.6 (136/86). This value represents the increased risk of mortality from all causes, for the unemployed seeking work, against the employed. The all cause mortality hides a wider range of SMRs for specific diseases. For all cancers it is 141, for respiratory disease 146, for lung cancer 175, and for suicide 241. One of the underlying problems of interpreting associations even when they are strong is that some other variable may actually be the determinant. In the case of unemployment it may be that the person became unemployed because they were sick.

Alternatively, it may be social class, income, or a combination of social variables. What Moser, Fox and Jones tried to do was to look at these SMRs again, and control for certain other variables.[3] The association between social class and health has been very well established since Farr's original work and records at Somerset House from 1837. People in social class I have a very different mortality experience from those in social class V. Figure 4 (page 132) shows the SMRs by social class for all men, for those unemployed seeking work, and for those unemployed seeking work standardised for social class. The SMRs for all men vary from 73 in social class I to 120 in social class V. In this case 120 to 73 represents a relative risk of 1.6 comparing social class V with social class I. The results are similar amongst the unemployed seeking work. The SMR ranges from 79 to 150 demonstrating again a significant social class gradient. The final column of the table shows the risk, standardised for social class. The increased risk of dying in social class I if you are unemployed is 103 which in fact is not significant. In social class IV it is 150 and in social class V 124. The average is 121. Standardising for social class reduces the excess mortality from 136 to 121. Again comparing the unemployed seeking work with the employed (SMR 86) the relative risk has been reduced from 1.6 to 1.4. This means that we still have an increased risk of 40 per cent for all causes. For specific causes, for example suicide, the SMR standardised for social class is still over 200.

Figure 4 Mortality 1971–1981 by social class of all men (aged 15–64 at death) and unemployed men seeking work in 1971 (aged 15–64 at death)

SOCIAL CLASS	SMR ALL MEN	SMR UNEMPLOYED SEEKING WORK	SMR UNEMPLOYED SEEKING WORK STANDARDISED FOR SOCIAL CLASS
I	73	79	103
II	78	109	139
IIIn	98	113	116
IIIm	94	123	132
IV	103	255	250
V	120	150	124
TOTAL	100	136	121

From Moser, Fox and Jones 1984

Almost without exception, studies of unemployment in this country have looked at male unemployment and have ignored the problem of female unemployment. The closest approximation we have of the effect on women is from studies of wives of unemployed men. Moser, Fox and Jones found that the wives of unemployed men followed for ten years had an SMR from all causes of 120 and of 160 for suicide.

Biological gradient

The concept of biological gradient is well understood in the field of pharmacology where it tends to be described in terms of dose response. This implies that the more you are exposed to a causative agent the more likely you are to suffer an effect. Returning to the example of smokers, Doll and Hill showed that the increased risk if you smoke up to 14 a day, 15–24 and over 25 a day was 8 times, 20 times and 32 times higher than amongst non-smokers.[5] The more you smoke the more likely you are to die of lung cancer. The unemployment literature is relatively weak in this regard but recent studies, including that of Platt and Kreitman in Edinburgh, have looked at the length of unemployment. Amongst those who were unemployed for less than 4 weeks, 5–26 weeks, 27–52 weeks or more than 52 weeks, the relative risk of para-suicide was 8.8, 5.4, 10.4 and 18.9. The relationship may not be simple. It suggests a possible 'U' shaped curve with an early increased risk during the first four weeks. The relative risk is highest amongst those unemployed for more than one year, and the value of 18.9 cannot easily be dismissed.

Consistency

This implies that a whole set of studies over different periods of time in different places performed by different researchers have revealed similar results. Consistency has certainly been the case in the field of unemployment and health. Much of the work was done in the 1920s and 1930s[6–10] but there has been a resurgence of interest during the last few years.[11–13] These studies, of which there are now several hundred, have adopted a variety of different strategies. They include case control and cohort studies, studies of individuals and aggregates across countries. In summary they all broadly agree on the association between unemployment and ill health, both in terms of mortality and morbidity.

Relationship in time

It is difficult to separate out the effects of poor health on employment and unemployment on future health. It is said by many of the critics of the unemployment and health hypothesis that people are unemployed because they are ill. They are the ones who cannot find jobs in the first place. They are the ones who are the first to be laid-off. It has been recognised for a long time that studies of the employed must take account of the selection bias, known as the healthy worker effect. Fagin and Little selected men from the DHSS cohort of 2300 men who first registered as unemployed in the autumn of 1978.[14] Their criteria for selection required that the man had been in continuous employment throughout 1977 and had not lost time through sickness or ill health prior to being laid-off. Analysis of their small subset suggested that unemployment came first and sickness second. The National Training Survey also concluded that this was the more important order of events.[15] Nevertheless the whole question of time relationship, which came first the chicken or the egg, is unsatisfactory in this field and few studies have given entirely convincing answers.

Plausibility

Plausibility is perhaps the most difficult of the criteria because what is implausible today, may in fact be very plausible in ten years time. For it to be understandable we need to be able to believe in a mechanism. Perhaps the most persuasive of the several possible mechanisms is that proposed by Jahodah.[12] In trying to understand the effect of unemployment she first put forward the reasons why people were employed. The primary reason was to earn a living. With loss of employment the primary loss was income and all the things that go with it. It is not difficult to relate resources to health. If you do not have sufficient resources to clothe yourself, to heat your house or indeed to have a house at all, then you are much more likely to die or become ill than if you do have those things. Resources and mortality are very carefully and closely linked. She considered however that it was the secondary benefits of employment that were even more important than the primary one involving resources. She listed them as status, self-esteem, self-image, activity, the imposition of a time structure on the waking day and the working together for some corporate goal. It is the loss of these that seem to be so damaging. If one loses the imposed timetable it is possible to lie in bed all day with nothing to do and that in itself can be very destructive. It may sound marvellous to those who, like university lecturers, yearn for a sabbatical year. Some indeed find it a marvellous experience; others are completely lost. They do not know what to do, and do nothing. The question of contact and shared experiences outside the family is probably more important. People also need to be valued; their status and self-esteem are important. If all these secondary benefits of employment are lost then people suffer. Perhaps a parallel example from the bereavement literature can best illustrate the effect of loss.[16] The loss of a spouse or loss of a father or mother, or a son or daughter, results in an increased risk of dying. The life events literature suggests that other major changes put great stress on an individual's health. So in the case of unemployment the loss of resources and the other benefits of employment put great stress on the individual and the effect is an increase in mortality and morbidity.

Experimental evidence

At the animal level, studies of social behaviour would lend support to the view that isolation has an adverse effect on health. In the absence of real experiments, epidemiologists have had to rely on quasi experiments. The closure of whole factories has been studied[17,18] but rarely for long enough or with adequate controls to be able to draw firm conclusions.

Conclusion

Taken together, the various criteria point firmly to the conclusion that unemployment causes ill health. The evidence is, in some cases, equivocal and in others circumstantial. However this evidence can be compared with that linking cholera and infection from the water supply. John Snow[19], a footleather epidemiologist, studied the number of people who died of cholera, who took their water from one supply system, or another. He found that there was an increased risk of about 8 times. Now he was not able to show a dose response relationship between the two – water supply and cholera. He was able to show a time relationship, but in terms of consistency he only had one study. When it came to plausibility he was laughed at. The concept – that is, in the 1850s – that there might be something in the water which would lead to the deaths of hundreds of people was thought to be outrageous and intrinsically unlikely. Thought at that time was not based on a microscopic view of organisms. If he had been an academic epidemiologist, he would have done what many of the epidemiologists and researchers in Britain are doing now in relation to unemployment which is calling for more evidence, more studies in depth, with better controls. What he actually did was to remove the handle of the parish pump so that people could not drink the water. Now that act of supreme civil disobedience could be called a community medicine approach to problem solving. In the unemployment debate the evidence is good but not conclusive. But on balance I think it is certainly good enough for us to say that there is a cause and effect relationship. It is not a huge difference, perhaps a 20 per cent increased risk of dying but, nevertheless, this amounts to thousands of people. It is not just a question of dying; there are increases in morbidity across a wide range of illnesses.

The issue for community medicine is how to minimise these adverse consequences. One approach is to treat the disease. It is possible, though difficult, to reduce the economic impact on the unemployed. In 1911 the National Insurance Act gave doctors the power to prescribe for the first time what was in effect money when they certified sickness. Now the doctors' involvement is likely to be limited to giving advice on entitlement for social benefits, an area about which many doctors are particularly ill informed. Another approach would be to try and help minimise the effects of the loss of secondary consequences. This means organising, or helping people themselves to organise, activities. People need a place where they can meet friends and do things that they enjoy. Such local initiatives have only a limited impact on the real problem.

I think the main challenge for doctors in community medicine is to tackle the root cause which is the high level of unemployment. This primary preventive approach will put doctors in conflict with the government. For those who claim to be concerned with the public health it will involve the development of advice which seeks to change existing policy. Nevertheless it would appear to be the only way of removing the handle of the parish pump.

Notes and references

1 S Platt and N Kreitman. Trends in parasuicide and unemployment among men in Edinburgh 1968–82. British Medical Journal, 289, 1984, pages 1029–1032.

2 A J Fox and P O Goldblatt. Longitudinal study: sociodemographic mortality differentials. London, HMSO, 1982. (Series LS no 1)

3 K A Moser, A J Fox and D R Jones. Unemployment and mortality in the OPCS longitudinal study. Lancet, II, 8 December 1984, pages 1324–1329.

4 S C Farrow. Monitoring the health effects of unemployment. Journal of the Royal College of Physicians, 17, no 2, pages 99–105.

5 R Doll and A B Hill. A study of the aetiology of carcinoma of the lung. British Medical Journal, 2, 1952, pages 1271–1286.

6 M Lazarsfeld-Jahoda and H Zeisl. Psychologische Monographien, 5, 1933, page 123.

7 E W Bakke. The unemployed man. London, Nisbet, 1933.

8 The Pilgrim Trust. Men without work. London, Macmillan, 1938.

9 P Eisenberg and P F Lazarsfeld. Psychological Bulletin, 35, 1938, page 358.

10 H Singer. Unemployment and Health. Pilgrim Trust Unemployment Enquiry Interim Paper, 4, 1937.

11 P B Warr. Some studies of psychological well-being and unemployment. Memo 43, Sheffield, Social and Applied Psychology Unit, 1981.

12 M Jahoda and H Rush. Work, employment and unemployment. University of Sussex, Science Policy Research Unit, 1980.

13 M H Brenner. Mortality and the national economy: a review, and the experience of England and Wales, 1936–76. Lancet, II, 1979, pages 568–573.

14 L Fagin and M Little. Unemployment and health in families: case interviews based on family studies: a pilot study. London, DHSS, 1981.

15 D Metcalf and S J Nickell. Notes on the incidence of unemployment and sickness spells of 3 months or more 1965–1975. CLE Working Paper, 1979, page 72.

16 C M Parkes. Bereavement: studies of grief in adult life. Harmondsworth, Penguin, 1975.

17 S Westin and D Norum. Nar sardinfabrikken Nellegges. University of Bergen, Institutt for Hygiene og Sozialmedisin, 1977.

18 L Iverson and H Klausen. Lukningen af Nordhavns-Vaerflet. Kobenhavns Universitet, Institut for Social Medicin, 1981.

19 J Snow. On the mode of communication of cholera. 1855. (Reprinted 1936, Cambridge, Mass)

RESPONSIBILITY: LAW, MEDICINE OR MORALS?

Nicola Lacey

The concept of responsibility is one which is appealed to in a wide variety of spheres of discourse. Notably, it forms an important part of the linguistic currency of moral philosophers and criminal lawyers as well as helping to shape what we might call common sense judgements about the status to be accorded to the actions of individuals. In this paper I shall be concerned with the question of whether the conceptions of responsibility appealed to in these various areas are one and the same, particularly in respect of whether they serve similar functions in the different areas. In particular I shall be addressing the question of how far it is realistic and appropriate for the legal system to expect doctors and psychiatrists to come into court and give evidence geared towards attribution of the criminal lawyer's conception of responsibility. This is the case when they are called upon to give evidence relevant to a finding of 'abnormality of mind' such as to result in a 'substantial impairment of mental responsibility' for the purposes of making out the defence of diminished responsibility under section 2(1) of the Homicide Act 1957.

The first part of the paper will investigate the nature and extent of the connection between philosophical conceptions of responsibility and those used by the criminal law, and will raise the question of whether recent developments in the law relating to *mens rea* have disturbed the traditional principle of criminal liability as based on moral capacity-responsibility. The second part of the paper will consider the extent to which the differing practical orientations of lawyers on the one hand and doctors on the other renders futile or inappropriate the enterprise of eliciting medical judgements framed in terms of legal conceptions. I shall also consider whether the changing basis of the legal conception of responsibility will either aggravate or mitigate the situation.

Moral responsibility and criminal liability

The question of the moral basis of criminal liability, encompassing questions not only of responsibility but also of the proper limits of the criminal law and of the justification for punishment, has received much attention from lawyers and philosophers alike. I shall not here be concerned with the fundamental philosophical issue of whether individuals can ever be said to be responsible for their actions, in the sense of having some measure of free will, or whether all our actions are in fact causally determined. I shall take as my starting point the criminal law's working presupposition of the possibility of responsibility, and consider the rationales which have been proposed for what has become known as the '*mens rea* principle': the presumption that, unless the contrary intention is made clear in the statutory formulation, some measure of responsibility for the *actus reus* of an offence, in the sense of intention, recklessness or, sometimes, negligence, will have to be proved in order to secure a conviction. The rationale for this principle has been most lucidly and persuasively explained by H L A Hart[1] as resting on the moral notion of capacity-responsibility combined with a principle of fairness. Unless a defendant is responsible for her action in the sense of both understanding its nature and having the opportunity to do otherwise than she does, it would be unfair to blame, let alone punish, her for what she has done. The value of the principle of fairness is fleshed out by Hart in terms of the harms of uncertainty and unpredictability which would be engendered should individuals not be able to plan their lives so as to avoid the intervention of the criminal law[2], as would be the case if it punished them for mere accidents. But it is clear that Hart does not mean his defence of the principle to rest on its utilitarian recommendations: he bases his argument on the widely shared intuition that, apart from exceptional circumstances (such as instances of strict liability in criminal law), it would be wrong to sacrifice the value of fairness embodied in the principle of not blaming people except for actions which proceed from informed choices, simply because the balance of utilities comes out in favour of the sacrifice. These commonsense intuitions are nicely brought out by Hart in his example of our differing reactions to being jostled in a crowded place:[3] if the action is deliberate, we feel anger and even affront; if it is accidental, minor irritation or simple tolerance; if negligent, something in between.

The difficulty with both the moral thesis offered by Hart and its potential as a rationalisation of the criminal law is quite simply that our intuitions on the subject are complex and often not consistent. Thus some stronger basis will have to be found to ground the moral principle, and even if this can be done successfully, the rationalisation must become a prescription, given the clear fact that the current criminal law reflects the complexity of our intuitions. For example, Clarkson and Keating[4] point out that our reactive attitude to a negligent or drunken driver alters dramatically according to whether she actually has an accident or not. Although the drunken or careless state may be equal in each case, our instinct is to blame to a greater degree the driver who actually injures or kills, despite the fact that, given the careless or drunken state, the harm was caused accidentally. This is reflected in the law by the fact, for example, that the offence of reckless driving is punishable less severely than that of causing death by reckless driving[5] and, conversely, by the practice of punishing attempts less severely than completed crimes. The harm caused appears to influence legal sentencing judgements in as important a way as the degree of responsibility, even to the extent of grounding assertions of punishment-worthiness in the absence of capacity-responsibility in any real sense.

Hart provides a spirited defence of negligence liability as a genuine form of *mens rea* liability[6] on the basis that, so long as the defendant had a real opportunity to reach the standard of care, to behave as a reasonable man or woman would have behaved, then she can be said to be behaving responsibly. But just what is it that she is responsible *for*? On the traditional theory, it cannot be said without distortion, for example, that she is responsible for running into the lamp-post and damaging it: it would be more accurate to say that she was responsible for her failure to attain the required standard of care, the actual outcome of that failure being, strictly speaking, fortuitous. In sum, two things seem to be clear. First, the law *does* make the trade-offs between the responsibility principle and utilitarian gains such as general deterrence in just the way in which Hart claims to be ruled out, normatively speaking, in more than just exceptional cases. Secondly, at least some of the cases in which it makes such trade-offs seem to be based not on mere expediency but on a conviction that the law is justified in reflecting certain widespread reactive attitudes concerning the extent to which harm caused affects the blameworthiness of actions independently of the responsibility principle.

The suspicion that the factors I have referred to undermine the potency of the traditional theory of responsibility as a rationalisation of the principles of criminal liability in English law, is reinforced by certain recent developments in the common law, notably by the decision of the House of Lords in *Caldwell*.[7] In that case their Lordships decided that the common law concept of recklessness encompassed not only the state of mind of foreseeing a risk and going ahead regardless of it but also that of failure to appreciate a risk in circumstances in which a reasonable person would have done so. Since this conception of recklessness extends at least to a wide variety of statutory offences[8] it is clear that the greater part of the criminal law now consists of offences which can be committed not merely with the traditional forms of subjective *mens rea* but also by means of what is essentially negligence. Thus if the argument that negligence liability cannot be accommodated within the traditional principle of responsibility except by means of distortion is correct, it is clear that the traditional theory no longer serves to rationalise the basis of liability in the greater part of the criminal law. The orthodox practice of regarding instances of strict liability as exceptional (questionable in itself given the wide range of cases in which the *mens rea* requirement has been held not to run to all the elements of the *actus reus*[9]) can no longer be maintained in the light of this recent development. We are faced with the stark alternatives of either condemning those developments and hanging on to the responsibility principle, or seeking some other rationalisation for the existing law (bearing in mind, of course, that not all the developments may be justifiable either in the sense of being capable of rationalisation within a coherent descriptive theory of the criminal law or at the fully normative level). Even if we do retain our normative commitment to the responsibility principle, the enterprise of trying to elicit the reasons for the law's development away from it may well seem worthwhile nevertheless.

Perhaps the alternative Humean conception of responsibility which has recently been reassessed by Michael Bayles[10] may prove to be of help. According to this conception, assertions of responsibility are based upon judgements about the *character* of the agent: actions for which we hold a person fully responsible are those in which her usual character is centrally expressed. Thus, to give some examples from the criminal law, actions performed as a result of provocation, duress or temporary mental incapacity will be regarded as non- or partially responsible. The finding of *mens rea*, such as intention or recklessness on the character model, provides an important piece of evidence from which the existence of character responsibility may be inferred, given that single acts do not always indicate settled dispositions. Whilst this model seems to give an adequate rationale for some of the most familiar excuses, it also serves to point up some possible reasons for the law's ambivalence concerning others. Actions performed by a person suffering from a long-term mental incapacity, whilst they call for a different reactive response in terms of traditional conceptions of blameworthiness, still appear to call for some controlling intervention on the part of the state. For since the action cannot be said to be a mere aberration on the part of the accused, the risks of repitition may be high. Hence, in our current criminal law, although the insanity defence absolves the defendant from any theoretical criminal liability, it does not remove her from the ambit of legal intervention of a radical kind. Similarly, although more controversially, a person who claims that her offence was committed because she was labouring under a mistake of fact may be regarded in a different light according to whether the mistake is one which the jury thinks any reasonable person might have made or not: if not, perhaps this is a person who systematically makes unreasonable mistakes, causing danger to the interests of others. The link with a possible rationalisation for negligence liability is obvious.

The rejoinder of the supporter of the traditional theory of responsibility to these suggestions is obvious enough. In her sense, we are not responsible for our characters, and to base our legal conception of responsibility on such a footing would smack of illicitly blaming people for what they are, which they cannot help, rather than for what they do, which they often can – a practice often roundly condemned in text on criminal law and, indeed, in judicial rhetoric. The objection flows from the way in which the character conception severs the link between voluntariness and responsibility, as is well illustrated by our earlier discussion of the implications of the conception for mentally disordered offenders.

This is not the place to conclude this very complex debate at the normative level. At the level of producing a descriptive theory of the criminal law, I would argue that the merit of the character conception of responsibility is that it serves to highlight the fundamentally important practical orientation of the criminal law as a form of social control; that it seeks to reduce, by means of prohibition, conviction and punishment, certain unwanted forms of behaviour. This essentially functionalist, forward-looking approach of the criminal law is reflected in its frequent departures from the traditional theory of responsibility and in its focus on harms caused and threatened (as in the case of the inchoate offences). But it would be wrong to concede that this model does not also have moral recommendations: it does not simply allow individual defendants to be sacrificed on the altar of general deterrence or public protection whatever the basis and antecedents of their *actus reus* may be. Instead of inquiring directly into a state of mind accompanying that *actus reus*, it asks a wider set of questions about the defendant herself and the extent to which the *actus reus* was a typical example of her behaviour, thus reflecting the reactive attitudes we express when we excuse someone's bad behaviour on the basis that it was 'out of character' or 'not like her' – reactive attitudes every bit as strong as those adduced by the traditional theory in support of its conception of responsibility. On that theory, it may well be true that we are not to blame for our characters. But the criminal law has to deal with us as we are, and given its task of helping to create the conditions for tolerable social existence, it is not open to it to excuse individuals for unavoidable characteristics which make them dangerous to others, at least to the extent of removing them from the ambit of criminal regulation completely.

This may appear to be a morally repugnant conclusion, but it can perhaps be seen in proportion with the help of some reflection on the extent to which luck and other unavoidable factors inevitably affect people's life chances in almost every area. Furthermore, although, as I have argued, there is a significant overlap between assertions of responsibility and assertions of blameworthiness, that overlap is limited. In other words, an ascription of character responsibility is *not* identical with an assertion of blameworthiness. This means that the character conception will not suffice as the central principle of responsibility in purely moral discourse: indeed it may well be that the capacity conception more nearly captures our intuitions at the moral level. The legal arena, however, displays special features which render appropriate a different conception of responsibility as one important determinant of criminal liability. These consist in the fact that, on the functionalist view of the criminal justice system which I have sketched, there is no automatic relationship between criminal conviction and moral culpability. Naturally, the contingent connection between the two fosters the tendency of judges, journalists and others to equate them: it is, however, an important part of my argument that such an equation is illicit. If this tendency could be reduced, the force of the traditionalist's objection to the character conception of responsibility as the basis for criminal liability would be substantially reduced.

Legal conceptions of responsibility and expert medical evidence

How far does the debate we have been discussing concerning different approaches to the legal conception of criminal responsibility bear upon the role of the expert medical witness in a criminal trial? The difficulties encountered by such witnesses have been the subject of much comment[11], and the reasons for their difficulties are easy to suggest, if harder to resolve. Perhaps one of the most graphic illustrations is that of the notorious Yorkshire Ripper case[12] in which the judge refused to accept the defendant's plea of diminished responsibility despite unanimous psychiatric evidence supporting it and the prosecution's willingness to accept it. This caused a major part of the trial to consist in a cross-examination of medical witnesses contending that Sutcliffe's state of mind at the time of the offences consisted in the substantial impairment of mental responsibility necessary to ground the defence.[13] The ultimate conviction of Sutcliffe for murder raised grave questions not only about the appropriateness of staging such medical arguments in the legal arena so as to deduce legal consequences from their outcome. It also raised questions about the extent to which policy considerations, such as the strong public feeling that Sutcliffe should be convicted as a murderer rather than a mere manslaughterer, should be allowed to subvert (largely in the guise of allegedly 'objective' legal judgements) the place of the defence of diminished responsibility in the criminal law. If Sutcliffe's testimony to the effect that he had been directed by voices to wage a campaign against prostitutes was to be believed, one wonders whether any case would satisfy the requirements of the defence in view of the fact that this apparently did not constitute a substantial impairment of responsibility.

I would argue that the clue to the reluctance of the court, the jury and indeed public opinion to allow Sutcliffe's plea is intimately connected with our generally complex and even confused attitudes to the notion of responsibility within the criminal law and indeed to the role of the criminal law in general. On the one hand, the traditional conception of responsibility is linked to the view of criminal conviction as reflecting culpability and expressing condemnation of a past action, and to the notion of criminal punishment as being observed. This deeply held attitude issues in a reluctance to see a defendant whose actions have caused grave harm and have outraged public sentiment being 'excused' in any way, despite the facts that a) this would not have reduced the law's capacity to intervene and control the defendant's future activities, a maximum life sentence being available for manslaughter; and b), paradoxically, that the conviction for murder may well not have been justified on a careful application of the very notion of responsibility which I have argued forms a large part of the basis for these strong reactive attitudes to do with desert.

Turning to the specific question of the position of the expert witness, attention to the traditional conception of criminal responsibility can, I would suggest, be shown to involve more serious problems than would a focus on the alternative character conception. This can best be brought out by reflecting on the differing practical orientations of doctors and of lawyers. The doctor, in making clinical judgements, at least in the sphere of practice, is directed in general to the practical question of what action should be taken to remedy or stabilise the patient's condition. Diagnosis, in other words, is practically important in that it leads to conclusions about proper treatment, at least in areas where medical knowledge is reasonably advanced. The lawyer's question about whether a defendant acted responsibly differs in a fundamental way in its orientation from this (admittedly simplistic) model of diagnosis leading to decisions about treatment. The exact nature of the decision in terms of its practical significance can be put in two competing ways, each consistent with the traditional conception. On the retributivist view, the 'diagnosis' of responsibility for the *actus reus* is both a necessary and a sufficient condition for the justifiability of punishment: the orientation here is exclusively 'backward-looking' in that the punitive response is geared only to desert for responsible actions in the past and not to any future benefits to be secured by the sanction. Thus, although the judgement of responsibility gives guidance about the proper punitive response in the sense that desert indicates not only that punishment is justified but also how much punishment may be inflicted, this guidance has no reference whatsoever to any question about consequences (at least in an ordinary, as opposed to a metaphysical sense) sought to be attained.

On the Hartian view, the judgement of responsibility operates as a necessary but not a sufficient condition for punishment; the general aim of punishment is said to be forward-looking, pursuing such goals as general deterrence or social protection. The way in which this model departs from the medical one differs from the way in which the purely retributive view does, but there is nevertheless a sharp distinction to the medical model in the fact that the judgement of responsibility itself is seen as being separate and distinct from any forward-looking question about what ought to be done with the offender.

In the retributivist case, then, no truly forward-looking question arises, due to the hypothesis that some relationship may be ascertained between culpability and desert of a particular penalty. This somewhat mysterious process of reasoning clearly has little in common with the practical question being addressed by a doctor when she makes a decision on treatment in the light of diagnosis. On the Hartian model, the decision about how to treat an offender after conviction does comprise questions about what effects are sought to be created (although of course they will not be exclusively effects on the offender herself), but it differs from the medical model in that the 'diagnosis' of responsibility operates only as a threshold and does not contribute to the sentencing decision (except in a rather indeterminate way in the area of upper limits) in the direct way in which medical diagnosis contributes to the practical decision about treatment. Thus, when a doctor is asked to come into court and advise the judge and jury on the state of the defendant's mind in terms of 'mental responsibility' at the time of the offence, she is being asked to perform a practical task which is very different from anything else within her experience. She is being asked to judge, in an apparently objective way, what was a defendant's state of mind at a time in the past, totally independently of any practical question about what should be done with that defendant (at least in theory) – a decision very unlike any which she would make in her own practice. I have added the words 'at least in theory' because, as the Sutcliffe case so clearly shows, considerations about the effects of a particular conviction do in practice affect and distort the way in which the court will respond to medical evidence. But this effect is covert. The doctor cannot explicitly appeal to such considerations nor can the court acknowledge their existence: things proceed on the basis of the theoretical position which I have described.

Another good illustration of the interaction in practice of question of responsibility and questions of consequences to be found in the law reports is the case of *Sullivan*[14], an epileptic who pleaded the defence of non-insane automatism to the offence of assault occasioning actual bodily harm under section

47 of the Offences Against the Person Act 1861 committed whilst he was in the throes of a fit. The court rejected the plea and stated that the only defence available was that of insanity, on the legal basis that epilepsy was a factor which affected mental capacity within the definition of the M'Naghten rules[15] as springing from a 'disease of the mind' and thus could not also ground the defence of automatism. The true rationale of this decision lies, I would suggest, in the fact that a successful plea of automatism would have led to an acquittal and thus to the absence of power in the court to exercise any legal control over the defendant. The court felt that someone who, irrespective of culpability or responsibility in the traditional sense, presented a threat to social security should be subject to some measure of legal control. Under present legal arrangements, the only way in which the court could assume any power was by defining the mental incapacity as insanity. This, incidentally, gave rise to a withdrawal of the automatism defence and a plea of guilty to the offence charged, thus in fact cutting down the measure of control available to the court.

This case raises in a stark form the question of whether our legal arrangements would do better explicitly to acknowledge and accommodate the functionalist considerations which we have seen as influencing and indeed distorting the application of the law in the Sutcliffe and Sullivan cases, and to attempt to move gradually towards a general view of the criminal law as a consequence-oriented enterprise rather than as a system devoted to producing crude reflections of common moral judgements about blameworthiness, desert and culpability. I should like to suggest that the move in this direction has already begun, through the developments outlined in the previous section, and, incidentally, that a rationalisation of the basis of criminal liability through the character conception of responsibility would resolve at least one of the causes of difficulty for expert medical witnesses in criminal trials. I have already argued that the character conception of responsibility fits well with the criminal law's function of controlling certain forms of what is generally thought to be unacceptable behaviour in the social context, in that its identification of responsibility is centrally concerned with the typicality of the behaviour in question, which is in turn linked with judgements of the likelihood of repetition. This is not to say that this conception of responsibility is unrelated to reactive attitudes attributing blame: as we saw, the claim that a certain act was 'out of character' often is put as an absolving or excusing comment in the sphere of moral evaluation. But the link between blameworthiness and character responsibility is indirect and contingent rather than direct or conceptual. This is best illustrated by the case of the insane offender, who, on the character conception, is responsible for her offence despite the absence of either blameworthiness or capacity responsibility in the traditional sense. The character conception is thus concerned with the degree to which an action reflects the settled personality traits of the agent, and as such the question of responsibility becomes intimately linked with practical conclusions about what sort of response (in our case, the response of the criminal law) is justified and appropriate. This conception of responsibility does not operate as a mere threshold, a necessary condition for conviction, a side constraint on the pursuit of policy objectives; it acts instead as an integral part of the substantive justification for the intervention of the law and an important guide as to the form which that intervention should take. Its consequentialist orientation distinguishes it from the retributive model, and it avoids the two-stage procedure of treating the questions of conviction and sentence as subject to entirely different modes of reasoning characteristic of the Hartian model. It also separates more clearly than does the traditional conception the issues of legal and moral guilt.

The connection between these arguments and a partial resolution of the doctor's dilemma is, I hope, relatively clear. Let us imagine a system in which doctors were asked to advise the court on the question of the extent to which the offence represented a central expression of the offender's personality rather than a question about the state of mind with which an offence was committed. The practical point of the question would be the fundamental problem of what should be done with the offender – whether the law's coercive powers should be brought to bear in view of the risks presented by this individual to social safety. Surely this question would make a great deal more sense to doctors than does the present question. Naturally it will not preclude consideration of the defendant's state of mind; this will often be of great importance. But in making explicit the link between the issue of responsibility and the practical question of sentence, surely the analogy with the doctor's practical orientation of diagnosis and treatment will render the task more straightforward.

This can perhaps be best illustrated by looking at the effect such a mode of argument would have had in the Sutcliffe and Sullivan cases. In Sutcliffe's case, given the length of time over which his offences were committed, and his apparent lack of remorse, it would have been difficult to make out an argument that his behaviour was atypical in the sense of removing character responsibility. What if, however, medical evidence was that this behaviour resulted merely from an easily corrected chemical imbalance which could be treated by one permanently effective injection? It is easy to see that release following treatment would not be a realistic possibility given the outrage felt at Sutcliffe's offences: my own view is, however, that his imprisonment in such circumstances would not be justified on the basis of either the traditional or the character conceptions of responsibility. The best way forward in such a case would be to acknowledge that there are occasionally justifications for confinement (an example outside the criminal justice system would be that of quarantine and one inside it the present treatment of offenders who are insane within the M'Naghten rules) which do not depend on assertions of responsibility. To admit this openly and to clarify the circumstances in which such confinement is justifiable would be preferable to pretending that responsibility does exist. This is another situation in which our conclusion would be more acceptable if progress could gradually be made towards weakening the association in popular and indeed legal consciousness between legal and moral guilt. As I have already argued, focusing on the character conception as the peculiarly legal conception of responsibility will at least be of some help in that respect.

Turning to the Sullivan case, once again the importance of weakening the presumptive link between legal and moral blameworthiness is apparent. On the character conception, if Sullivan's epileptic fits frequently resulted in violent or other dangerous or threatening behaviour, then responsibility is established and forms the basis of an argument for some measure of intervention by the criminal law. This clearly does not entail moral culpability, nor does it follow that the law's intervention should be particularly intrusive: but its central functionalist rationale dictates at least some degree of control. Here too, the character conception seems to cast the doctor in a more familiar and appropriate role: that of advising on the appropriate response to a diagnosis, where that diagnosis consists in an assertion of responsibility which may sometimes concern a peculiarly medical judgement.

At this point it is necessary to emphasise the very considerable differences which exist between the approach which I have been advocating and the 'medical' or 'treatment' model proposed by Baroness Wootton[16], and roundly criticised by Hart among others.[17] The essence of Wootton's argument is that we should abandon the traditional model of crime and punishment and move to one in which a crime was merely regarded as a symptom of some social disorder or maladjustment. Thus the state's response should be framed in terms of treatment aimed at rehabilitation, and the existence of responsibility would merely be one extra symptom which would aid the court and those entrusted with the care of the offender in identifying the appropriate diagnosis and therapeutic programme. Several clear differences exist between this approach and the character responsibility approach. In the first place, the character approach does not purport to provide a unitary theory of state intervention in criminal cases. We have already seen in our discussion of the Sutcliffe case that there may exist other strong functionalist reasons for state intervention, even in the absence of responsibility in the character sense. Thus that responsibility is not a necessary condition for the exercise of legal control but merely one (albeit potent) indicator of the appropriateness of a regulatory response. In addition, there are certain functionalist aims, such as general deterrence, to which the identification of responsibility is not necessarily a relevant 'diagnostic' factor to be taken into account in fixing the level of the penalty.

Secondly, the existence of responsibility in the character sense does not entail that the state response should be of a reformatory nature; it might equally (and more probably, given the empirical research on the possibility of rehabilitation) be geared at social protection through incapacitation (which, of course, need not always be by means of incarceration). Thus a system incorporating the character responsibility model as a central element would not be subject either to the counter-arguments based on the empirical evidence that our capacity to rehabilitate is practically non-existent[18], or to the counter-argument that the concept of social health encapsulated in the treatment model embodies an unacceptable denial of the possibility of human capacity responsibility. Nor would the argument that that concept is inherently manipulable and renders the criminal justice system a more potent political tool against those who do not conform to the government's conception of the ideal citizen, be applicable to the character responsibility view. For the character conception makes no assumption about the general basis of human behaviour: the possibility of capacity responsibility is entirely consistent with it. The character model merely claims that capacity responsibility is not generally the relevant conception for the purposes of deciding whether criminal regulation should be applied.

Conclusion

This paper has ranged over a wide number of issues in a rather cursory way, and makes it particularly necessary to provide by way of conclusion a summarised statement of the claims and suggestions which I wish to make about the role of the character conception of responsibility. First of all, I regard as highly questionable two sorts of claim made for the traditional capacity conception of responsibility. The first is the claim that it is an entirely adequate principle from the normative point of view, which I have argued is doubtful because of its failure to reflect certain strong intuitions which we hold about the way in which culpability is affected by harm caused, independently of ascriptions of responsibility. The second is the dual claim that this conception provides an adequate and an appropriate rationalisation of the basis of criminal liability. At the descriptive level this is questionable in view of the large and significant area of offences of strict liability and negligence, and in view of recent developments in the area of recklessness. At the prescriptive level it is questionable because, even if the capacity conception did allow us accurately to reflect blameworthiness in every case, this is not the central role of the criminal law. I have argued that the criminal law is best understood in terms of its social functions of control and prevention (among others), and that this characterisation renders the capacity conception inappropriate as a *general* principle of criminal liability.

The character conception of responsibility, on the other hand, appears to provide one important set of explanations of existing legal principles of *mens rea*, mitigation, excuse and justification, and to provide a rationalisation which does not encounter the difficulties met by the capacity conception. For it makes no general assumption about blameworthiness, being consistent with both the functionalist basis of the criminal law and the existence of blameworthiness in individual cases. Indeed the existence of capacity responsibility will often be an important factor in assessing the presence or absence of character responsibility. Moreover, as in the Sutcliffe case, general beliefs in the existence of capacity responsibility and the retributive reactive attitudes which this engenders may be relevant to the justification of punishment, via some other element of the functionalist rationale of the system. Thus the character conception does not claim exclusivity in justifying criminal interventions: it does, however, claim to occupy a place of importance, especially in identifying the types of cases in which we regard it as necessary and acceptable to depart from the traditional model.

The claim which I have made about the relevance of this debate to the giving of medical testimony on the existence of responsibility is a tentative one, but I would suggest that two points can be supported. The first is a general observation about the danger of assuming a wide measure of interchangeability of apparently similar concepts referred to in a range of spheres of reasoning. Even in the legal and philosophical areas, as we have seen, several conceptions of responsibility are being appealed to, and these are reflected in a wide variety of ways in ordinary language discourse as well. Given this variety, it seems unwise to assume that a doctor asked to assess a defendant's behaviour in terms of responsibility will necessarily be able to meet that request in the terms in which it is intended.

The second point follows on from this one. The way in which we appeal to concepts in particular discourses is relative to the task in hand: in other words, the conception of responsibility appealed to will be relative to whether what is in issue is diagnosis and treatment, an attribution of moral blame, a criminal conviction, and so on. If the legal conception being appealed to in areas such as diminished responsibility is indeed the capacity conception, then the gap between the doctor's general practical orientation and that of the judgement she is asked to make in court, which has no reference to the issue of what would be a proper response to the responsible action, is very wide indeed. If, however, it is the character conception which is in play, the gap narrows considerably, and, whilst it could hardly be claimed that this will sweep aside all the difficulties which exist in the area of expert medical evidence and the role it should play in the criminal process, it does seem to solve some problems by rendering the evidential task and the doctor's usual orientation more consistent. This is, of course, not an argument in itself for adopting the character conception: it is merely a fortuitous side-benefit of adoption of that conception – although no less welcome for that.

Finally, I should like to make it clear that I do not claim to have presented anything approaching a full set of arguments for the claims which I have put forward: to do this would be the business of a much larger project. What I hope to have done is to have thrown out some ideas not only about the place of the concept of responsibility in the criminal process, and of medical evidence in helping to decide whether responsibility should be attributed, but also about the interrelationship between different conceptions within legal discourse and the possibility of their coexistence and consistency. I have also put forward and argued a view of the criminal process which will be controversial and which I have not been able fully to argue for here. Nor has the theory of punishment underlying my remarks been fully described let alone adequately defended. But I hope at least to have raised some questions which will be of interest to legal philosophers, lawyers and doctors, in small contribution to the lively debate which is growing up, happily, between the disciplines.

Notes and references

1 H L A Hart. Punishment and responsibility. Oxford, Oxford University Press, 1968, chapters 1, 7 and 9.
2 See 1 above, pages 22–23.
3 See 1 above, pages 182–183.
4 C M V Clarkson and H M Keating. Criminal law: text and materials. London, 1984, pages 357–361, chapter 9.
5 Parliament. Road Traffic Act, 1972. London, HMSO, 1972, sections 1 and 2. (See Glanville Williams. Textbook of criminal law, second edition. London, Stevens, 1983, pages 313–321)
6 See 1 above, chapter 6.
7 (1982) AC 341.
8 For example, offences of criminal damage under the Criminal Damage Act, 1971, and of reckless driving under the Road Traffic Act, 1972. (See *Lawrence* (1982) AC 510)
9 Examples would be the offences of assault occasioning actual bodily harm under section 47 of the Offences Against the Person Act, 1861, for which *mens rea* is required as to the assault but not as to the harm, and of assaulting or obstructing a police constable in the execution of his duty under section 51 of the Police Act, 1964, in which *mens rea* need not run to the fact of the victim being a police constable. (See Williams, Textbook of Criminal Law (5 above), pages 191, 200, 929–930)
10 Michael Bayles. Character, purpose and criminal responsibility: 1 Law and philosophy, 1982, page 1.
11 For example, Dell. Criminal Law Review, 809, 1982; and Murder into manslaughter: the diminished responsibility defence in practice. Oxford, Oxford University Press, 1984.
12 *R v Sutcliffe* (1981): the Court of Appeal's refusal of leave to appeal was reported in The Times, 23 May 1982.
13 Williams. Textbook of Criminal Law (see 5 above), page 689.
14 (1983) 3 WLR 123.
15 10 Cl & F 200; 8 ER 718 (1843).
16 Baroness Wootton. Social science and social pathology, 1959; Crime and the criminal law, 1963.

17 See 1 above, chapters 7 and 8.
18 R Martinson. What works? – questions and answers about prison reform. The Public Interest, Spring 1974.

PARENTS, CHILDREN AND MEDICAL TREATMENT: THE LEGAL ISSUES

Brenda Hoggett

Introduction

The case of *Gillick v West Norfolk and Wisbech Area Health Authority and the Department of Health and Social Security* concerned whether a girl under 16 could lawfully be given contraceptive advice or treatment (including abortion) without her parents' consent. Mrs Gillick sought two declarations: the first, to the effect that DHSS guidance suggesting that in exceptional circumstances this might be done was 'unlawful and wrong'; the second, to the effect that any doctor or other professional person employed by the health authority might not give such advice or treatment to any of Mrs Gillick's children under the age of 16 without her prior knowledge and consent. Such declarations were refused by the High Court[2], granted by the Court of Appeal[3], and refused once more by a majority of three to two in the House of Lords.

Of all the judges who heard the case, only the two dissentients in the House of Lords based their reasoning on the particular nature of the treatment involved, and they differed from one another. Lord Brandon thought that providing such advice or treatment for a girl under 16 was so contrary to public policy as to be unlawful, and possibly criminal, whether or not there was parental consent. Lord Templeman thought that this was a particular form of treatment to which a girl under 16 was not competent to consent, and thus, subject to a few exceptions[4], only her parents could do so for her.

For all the other judges, however, the legal principles governing the relationship between parents, children and professionals applied equally to all forms of advice and treatment.

They are also relevant, not only to the case where a child under 16 wishes to have the treatment but the parent does not wish her to do so, but to the reverse situation, where the parent wishes the child to have treatment which the child does not want or which other people consider to be contrary to her welfare.

The best example of the latter situation in English law is the case of *Re D (a minor) (wardship: sterilisation)*.[5] Where a mother and paediatrician wished an 11-year-old girl with Sotos' syndrome to be sterilised, whereas those responsible for her education did not. Another example, which has already caused concern in the United States and is beginning to do so here, particularly with the development of private sector clinics specialising in adolescent behaviour disorders, is the so-called voluntary hospitalisation of children for treatment for mental disorder. In the American case of *Parham v JR*,[6] a child was admitted to a psychiatric hospital at the request of his mother when he was only six. He had already been expelled from school as uncontrollable and the diagnosis was a 'hyperkinetic reaction to childhood', but there had been only two months' outpatient treatment before his mother asked for his indefinite admission. Another child in the same case had been removed from his parents at the age of three months because of their neglect, but had had seven foster placements before his admission at the age of seven with a diagnosis of borderline mental handicap and an 'unsocialised, aggressive reaction to childhood'.

In the United States, such cases have to reconcile the constitutionally protected liberty interest of the child[7] with the equally protected commitment to the privacy and autonomy of the family. The end result was that the children did have a liberty interest which required protection from unwarranted invasions by the state, but that the independent judgement of the hospital superintendant was sufficient safeguard. Parents could generally be presumed to be acting in the best interests of their children, and safeguards which required formal adjudication would tend to exacerbate rather than heal family conflicts. In this country, we have no such principles entrenched in law, but the issues still concern the reconciliation of the rights of children as individuals with the so-called rights of parents, and in particular the extent to which it may be presumed, in the absence of legislation or litigation to the contrary, that a parent is acting in the best interests of a child.

Mental hospitalisation is a particularly good example of a situation in which a parent may well not be acting in the child's best interests.[8] Parents may turn to psychiatric treatment for a child in order to solve a problem which could be at least as much of their own making as of the child's. If their action results in the removal of the child, this may be of benefit to them, whether or not it also benefits the child. This is a particular risk where the child's behaviour is delinquent and an explanation based on mental disorder is less stigmatising for the family than one based on lack of control or criminal propensities. In other cases, the child's presence or behaviour may be seen by the parents as the cause of problems in the home which in fact stem from other causes, particularly where there is marital disharmony. Parents under stresses of this sort will be less able to assess the position realistically than they will in the case of ordinary physical disorders and even then objectivity will be impossible. Very similar arguments can apply to parental attitudes towards contraception and abortion, as these too are inextricably linked with the parents' own relationship with their children and their approach to exercising control.

The doctor's position is also much more difficult than in the case of ordinary physical disorders. Where the parent wants treatment for the child which the child does not want, the doctor is expected to safeguard the interests of the child by deciding whether to give or withhold the treatment. This is not easy, for the doctor is bound to rely upon the parents' accounts when eliciting the facts, especially where the child is very young. He may well have divided loyalties and, like many social workers, a very proper concern for the family as a whole in addition to the welfare of the individual child. There may be a tendency to over-diagnosis based on caution, although this appears to be a transatlantic phenomenon, and he may not have the time or the inclination to consult others involved. The child may already come bearing the label of one for whom others have not found the answer. Hospital staff cannot be expected to detect every mistaken judgement made earlier in a case, any more than the gynaecologist who agreed to sterilise the girl in *Re D* could be expected to assess much more than the gynaecological considerations when both the mother and the paediatrician wanted it done. In the last analysis, however, the doctor or other professional who believes that treatment is not in the child's best interests can protect the child's welfare by refusing to carry it out.

On the other hand, where the child wants treatment which the parent does not want her to have, the doctor who believes that the treatment is in her best interests has no such easy solution. It is a question of choosing between the rights of the child and the rights of the parent. Until the *Gillick* case, there were two competing methods of analysing the legal issues and little attempt at reconciling them. One method was adopted in the High Court, another in the Court of Appeal, and a synthesis was achieved in the House of Lords, although not, as we shall see, a complete one.

Children's rights

The first analysis starts from the proposition that hospital admission and medical treatment are potential invasions of clearly recognised rights of the patient herself. They dictate where she shall live and entail contact with her person for the purposes of treatment or care. If done without her consent or other lawful justification (such as statutory authority in the case of a compulsory admission under the procedures laid down in the Mental Health Act 1983) they will constitute a trespass to her person, no matter how carefully they have been carried out. They may give rise to an action for damages, or in some cases a prosecution, and a person unlawfully imprisoned may seek release through habeas corpus.

Modern learned literature, like the High Court in *Gillick* has tended to use this approach.[9] It has assumed that parental consent is required, not because the treatment would otherwise be an invasion of the rights of the parent, but because it would otherwise be an invasion of the rights of the child. The laws of tort and crime clearly protect the rights of children as much as those of adults. They may sue or prosecute for their injuries, including those caused by their parents. The main object of such laws is to protect people from harm, from having bodies less perfect than those with which they started out, but 'a citizen can be wronged without being harmed'[10] for otherwise medical treatment which is intended to do, and does do, nothing but good could be carried out without any consent at all. It is the patient who has the right to choose between the risks of treatment and the risks of non-treatment.

The English courts have not adopted the transatlantic concept of informed consent. Hence consent to treatment may be *real*, and thus a good defence to trespass, provided that the patient understands in broad terms what is proposed and agrees to it.[11] There is then no question of liability in damages unless the patient suffers harm. If the harm comes about because of negligence in diagnosis or carrying out the treatment, then there will be liability in the usual way. But the patient may suffer harm because one of the risks involved in the treatment itself does in fact materialise, even though all possible care has been taken. The only way in which there can be liability in such a case is where the patient shows, first, that the doctor was negligent in giving her advice about the treatment, and secondly, that had she been properly informed, she would not have given her consent at all, so that the harm she has suffered can clearly be said to have been caused by the negligent advice. The question of the standard to be applied in judging whether or not advice is negligent has given rise to great difficulty, and differing views were expressed in the House of Lords in the leading case of *Sidaway v Board of Governors of the Bethlem Royal Hospital and the Maudsley Hospital*.[12] The majority adopted the standard of the medical profession itself, so that a doctor would not be negligent if he acted in accordance with a practice accepted as proper by a body of responsible and skilled medical opinion[13], although in some case the disclosure of a particular risk might be 'so obviously necessary to an informed choice on the part of the patient that no reasonably prudent medical man would fail to make it'.[14]

For the purposes of the present discussion, the approach adopted by English law to issues of consent lends force to the analysis used in the High Court in *Gillick*. If a consent is real provided that the patient understands in broad terms what is proposed and agrees to it, then logically the capacity required of the patient to give that consent should not be great. A child who is capable of understanding the proposed treatment in such terms should be able to give her own consent.[15] Then if proper care is taken in advising and carrying out that treatment none of the child's rights have been infringed. The whole question becomes one of the child's own individual capacities, although it may well be that this is subject to the overriding consideration of the child's best interests, so that a child cannot validly consent to something which is not for her own good (such as the donation of blood or, in most cases, organs for transplant).

Statute supports this to some extent. Section 131(2) of the Mental Health Act 1983 provides for the informal admission to hospital for treatment for mental disorder of any child of 16 or over who is capable of expressing her own wishes, 'notwithstanding any right of custody or control vested by law in his [her] parent or guardian'. Section 8(1) of the Family Law Reform Act 1969 provides that the consent of a child of 16 to any surgical, medical or dental treatment 'shall be as effective as it would be if he [she] were of full age' and that if she consents it is unnecessary to obtain the consent of a parent or guardian.

Neither suggests that chronological age is the sole test. The Mental Health Act only applies if the child is capable of expressing a wish and the Family Law Reform Act only renders the consent as effective as it would be if the child were 18. Both therefore admit the possibility that a 16- or 17-year-old will be incapable of validating the action proposed. It may be that the Mental Health Act test of capacity is rather lower than the other, possibly because the Family Law Reform Act encourages as much informal admission as possible, and may thus on occasions blur the distinction between the consenting and the unprotesting.

Similarly, neither act suggests that a child below 16 is automatically incapable. The Mental Health Act refers to the possibly conflicting right of the parents, but, as Lord Fraser pointed out in the House of Lords in *Gillick*, this has no bearing on the possible capacity of the child herself: the question is whether custody necessarily involves the right to veto treatment which the child herself wants. The Family Law

Reform Act is relevant, for section 8(3) provides that 'nothing in this section shall be construed as making ineffective any consent which would have been effective if this section had not been enacted'. Hence, as the majority found, this act was concerned to make a clear presumption in the case of 16- and 17-year-olds, but left the capacity of other children to be decided according to the pre-existing law.

The majority also found that a girl under the age of 16 has the capacity to consent to advice, examination and treatment, provided that she has sufficient understanding and intelligence to know what they involve. It was pointed out that there are many situations in which the law recognises that children have the capacity to make legally relevant decisions. They may consent to sexual intercourse so as to prevent its being rape:[16] hence the need to legislate for a special offence of unlawful sexual intercourse.[17] The House of Lords has recently said that they may consent to go with someone so as to prevent that being kidnapping:[18] the capacity to do so would depend upon the individual facts in each case, although some children would obviously be too young. They may make certain types of contract.[19] They could consent to marriage, until legislation in 1929 which fixed the age of marriage in English law at 16.[20] They may give evidence on oath, provided that the court is satisfied that they understand the obligation to tell the truth[21], and specific enquiry is unlikely to be made of children of 14 or more. From the age of ten they may be held responsible for almost any criminal offence, and from the age of 14 there is no presumption that they do not know that what they are doing is seriously wrong, as there is below that age.[22]

Indeed, it is likely that all five of their Lordships in *Gillick* took the same general view on this issue. Apart from the three who did so expressly, Lord Brandon said nothing about the capacities of children to consent, because he held that *no one* could license this particular form of treatment for a girl under 16; but it was he who gave the leading speech in the kidnapping case referred to earlier.[23] Lord Templeman expressly accepted that 'a doctor may lawfully carry out some forms of treatment with the consent of an infant patient and against the opposition of a parent based on religious or any other grounds'. His point was simply that 'as the law now stands an unmarried girl under 16 is not competent to decide to practise sex and contraception'.[24]

They might also have agreed upon a quite stringent test of competence to be applied in deciding whether a particular child has the capacity to consent to a particular form of treatment. All agreed that it depends upon the nature of the treatment and the age and understanding of the child: Lord Templeman, for example, had no doubt that an intelligent boy or girl of 15 could consent to the removal of tonsils or appendix. But both he and Lord Scarman talked in terms of the child being able, not only to understand in general terms what is proposed, but of having the maturity to understand the emotional and moral implications of treatment such as contraception. Lord Scarman also speaks of a child having 'sufficient discretion to enable him or her to make a *wise* choice in his or her own interests'. Lord Fraser simply talks of the child having sufficient understanding and intelligence to know what the treatment involves. The distinction between knowing what is involved and having the capacity to make a wise decision is an important one. In the case of an adult, it is axiomatic that understanding, not wisdom, is all that is required for a man may go to the devil if he chooses. Perhaps, in the case of a child, it is permissible to ask for more, on the ground that the 'first and paramount consideration' throughout the law is the welfare of the child herself, so that the only treatment which anyone may permit is that which will promote her welfare. That, in essence, was the view taken by the majority in *Gillick* of the circumstances in which a doctor might rely upon the consent of the child herself when giving contraceptive advice and treatment.

Parental rights

Unfortunately, the analysis based upon the rights of the child leaves obvious gaps. If the child does not have the capacity to consent to treatment, someone must be able, and indeed obliged, to make decisions for her. In general, this will be her parents. But is their authority limited to making decisions on behalf of an incapable child, of any age up to 18; or may they give an alternative consent even when the child is capable, thus either overriding her dissent or (which in practice may amount to the same thing but is in theory less extreme) allowing the treatment to proceed without consulting her at all; and may they veto a treatment to which the child has given a valid consent?

The Court of Appeal in *Gillick* based its decision upon the existence of a parental right of custody and control which continued up until the age of majority at 18, subject to specific exceptions (such as section 8(1) of the Family Law Reform Act 1969) or the order of a court. Parents undoubtedly do have some control and authority over their children, but the concept of parental *rights* has been increasingly challenged in the literature.[25] One difficulty is that of establishing anyone with the corresponding duty to respect the parents' rights and refrain from interfering with them. Parents (more specifically fathers of legitimate children) used to have rights of action against third parties who deprived them of the services of their children, but most such actions were abolished by the Law Reform (Miscellaneous Provisions) Act 1970[26] and the remainder by the Administration of Justice Act 1982.[27]

Another difficulty is that attempts by parents to take legal action to enforce their claims or wishes, whether against one another, or against the child, or against most third parties, will be judged according to the 'first and paramount consideration' of the child's own welfare.[28] The claims and wishes of parents are obviously relevant in deciding what will promote her welfare, but the majority of the House of Lords in the leading case of *J v C*[29] considered that they were only relevant to that extent, and not as a separate consideration in their own right; all the judges in that case held that there was now no presumption in favour of the claims of natural parents, so that in the end the decision had always to be governed by what would best promote the welfare of the child in the widest sense.

Furthermore, although the statutory powers of the courts to interfere with parental decisions at the instance of third parties, whether individuals[30] or local authorities[31], are limited by reference to criteria laid down in the statutes themselves, the power of the High Court to intervene to protect the welfare of children is almost entirely unlimited.[32] It is not confined to issues about where the child should live or who should have care of her, but may also be invoked for specific decisions, including whether she should have, or not have, a particular form of medical treatment, such as sterilisation.[33] Although such interventions are extremely rare, the fact that they are possible at all in English law must cast doubt upon the validity of any concept of parental rights in the usual sense of that term.

The only remedy which might be available to a parent to enforce those rights is the injunction or declaration, as sought in *Gillick*. Both are discretionary remedies and where they relate to the upbringing of a child they should be governed by the welfare principle.[34] Hence it was surprising that the Court of Appeal granted a declaration having the same effect as an injunction, with respect to individual children, without having any evidence that it was needed or as to what would be in the best interests of those children.[35] Furthermore, by declaring the DHSS guidance unlawful, they were effectively giving notice that doctors and other professionals must not treat or advise *other* children as to whose welfare there was no evidence at all.

The Court of Appeal placed heavy reliance upon the Children Act 1975 which, for the first time, attempted a legislative explanation of certain concepts. 'Parental rights' is a phrase not frequently used in legislation, but it does appear in relation to their assumption by local authorities[36] and in the equality recently granted to mothers and fathers of legitimate children.[37] The 1975 Act defines 'the parental rights and duties' as 'all the rights and duties which by law the mother and father have in relation to a legitimate child and his property'[38], which throws us back to the common law. It further defines 'legal custody' as 'so much of the parental rights and duties as relate to the person of the child (including the place and manner in which his time is spent)....'[39] The main object of this provision was to define the effect of a court order giving 'legal custody' to a third party, but the act is so drafted that it is clear that parents do have 'legal custody' until it is taken away from them.[40] Otherwise, the effect of the definition is simply to throw us back to 'parental rights' and then to the common law.

The common law has a long history, but the House of Lords went back only as far as Blackstone's *Commentaries* of 1765. He does not speak of the rights of parents, but of their powers and authority[41], and he analyses these as the necessary concomitant of their parental duties. The corresponding duty to respect parental authority is owed as much by the child herself as it is by third parties. The attraction of this analysis is that the child is not then regarded as a species of property over which the parents have rights, but a person in a legal relationship with her own parents. The parents have a duty to respect her right to an adequate upbringing and in return she has the duty to respect their right to control that upbringing. Hence, 'the duties of children to their parents arise from a principle of natural justice and retribution. For to those, who gave us existence, we naturally owe subjection and obedience during our minority, and honour and reverence ever after....' However, 'the power of parents over their children is derived from the former consideration, their duty'[42] and their authority is given them 'partly to enable the parent more effectively to perform his duty and partly as a recompense for his care and trouble in the faithful discharge of it'.[43] The majority of the House of Lords in *Gillick* expressly adopted Blackstone's view that parental powers and authority were only the necessary concomitants of their duties towards their children: his further idea that they were also a reward for carrying out those duties was rejected.

But for how long do the parents' power and authority last? It is not difficult to find judicial support for a power of control which lasts throughout minority; the best-known example of this is *Re Agar-Ellis*[44], in which a 17-year-old girl was prevented from seeing her mother by a father whose authority was upheld by the Court of Appeal. This was the view essentially taken by the Court of Appeal in *Gillick*.

An alternative view would see parental powers lasting only so long as the concomitant duties last. Certain duties, for example relating to the child's property or marriage[45], may last until 18. Other duties, at least insofar as they are defined by the criminal law, last only until 16: these include the duty to provide adequate food, clothing, housing and medical aid[46], and to see that their children are properly educated.[47] A dividing line of 16 would, of course, have left the *Gillick* decision untouched. But there was already Court of Appeal authority for a more flexible approach.

In *Hewer v Bryant*[48], Lord Justice Sachs had drawn attention to the strict position at common law: 'the power of physical control over an infant by a father in his own right *qua* guardian by nature ... was and is recognised at common law; but that strict power ... in practice ceases on their reaching years of discretion.'[49] This was a reference to the refusal of the common law courts to grant habeaus corpus to a father to force an unwilling child to return to his custody once the child had reached the 'age of discretion'. In 1860, this was apparently fixed at 14 for boys and 16 for girls.[50] Lord Justice Sachs went on to say that once these powers of coercion had gone, the parent might have to turn for help to the court (originally the Chancery Court, exercising its inherent powers to protect all minors, which are now exercised by the Family Division of the High Court). The court might use its greater powers in aid of the father, and in the 19th century it tended to do so without question, but they were greater powers than his and might be used in a different way if the welfare of the child required it.

Lord Denning in *Hewer v Bryant* had taken an even more robust view: 'I would get rid of the rule in *Re Agar-Ellis* and of the suggested exceptions to it. That case was decided in the year 1883. It reflects the attitude of a Victorian parent towards his children. He expected unquestioning obedience to his commands. If a son disobeyed, his father would cut him off with a shilling. If a daughter had an illegitimate child, he would turn her out of the house. His power only ceased when the child became 21. I decline to accept a view so much out of date. The common law can, and should, keep pace with the times. It should declare ... that the legal right of a parent to the custody of a child ends at the 18th birthday: and even up till then, it is a dwindling right which the courts will hesitate to enforce against the wishes of the child, and the more so the older he is. It starts with a right of control and ends with little more than advice.'[51]

The majority in *Gillick* expressly agreed with that: not only is *Re Agar-Ellis* 'remaindered to the history books' but the whole idea of a set 'age of discretion' for certain purposes is replaced by a more flexible view based upon the capacities of the individual child and the nature of the decision to be taken (although there will be some matters which are regulated by statute).

The underlying principle is that parental powers are derived from the parental duties of maintenance, protection and education, and exist only for as long as is necessary to enable these to be carried out; usually this will be only until the child reaches an age to be able to look after herself and make her own decisions. However, it is clear that certain parental powers do exist *up until* that time and the precise effect of this for third parties such as doctors and social workers may need careful thought.

Hence it was agreed on all sides that a doctor might provide advice and treatment without parental consent in an emergency. Lord Templeman said that a doctor might proceed where he 'believes the treatment to be vital to the survival or health of an infant and notwithstanding the opposition of a parent or the impossibility of alerting the parent before the treatment is carried out'. Lord Templeman was also prepared to include a parental abandonment or abuse of their child in the circumstances in which a doctor might give contraceptive advice or treatment to an under-age girl without their consent, and presumably other forms of treatment to children who are in fact incapable of taking their own decisions. The majority did not address themselves to the position where the child was incapable, although they might well have agreed with Lord Templeman.

Nor was there any discussion of the reverse situation, where the parents wish the child to have treatment which the child does not want: the obvious examples are the psychiatric treatment discussed earlier or the termination of a pregnancy which the girl wishes to proceed. However, the capacity to consent must logically include the capacity to dissent: if, then, parental control is diminished to the extent that the child herself has acquired capacity, the parents should have no power to insist. If, on the other hand, parental control exists for as long as it is necessary to perform parental duties, the power to insist that a child receives treatment which is medically advised in her own best interests might persist for as long as the parents have the duty to supply 'adequate medical aid', that is until 16. Logically, the first view is to be preferred: a duty to provide adequate medical aid does not necessarily import a power to force it upon a competent child who has rejected it. Their Lordships, however, relied upon the 'parental duty' approach to parental authority without discussing what would happen where everyone apart from a competent child was satisfied that a particular treatment was in her best interests. It is not quite good enough to answer that such a child cannot be forced to comply, at least without resort to legal proceedings such as wardship or care proceedings. Many people, including children, will do as they are told by people whom they believe have the right to tell them what to do. We still cannot be sure whether or not parents have that right, although it seems likely that they do not.

Conclusion

The argument in this paper has not been concerned with the particular issue of whether it is, or is not, wise to permit doctors and other professionals to give contraceptive advice and treatment to girls under 16 without their parents' consent. As the law now stands, this can only be done in an emergency or where the girl herself is competent to consent and in each case the treatment or advice is in her own best interests. Lord Fraser translated this into five requirements, for the doctor to be satisfied:

i. that the girl will understand his advice;
ii. that he cannot persuade her to inform her parents or to allow him to do so;
iii. that she is very likely to begin or continue having sexual intercourse whether or not she has contraceptive treatment;
iv. that unless she receives contraceptive advice or treatment her physical or mental health or both are likely to suffer; and
v. that her best interests require him to give her contraceptive advice, treatment or both without the parental consent.

It seems likely that these guidelines will be operated in future practice, unless and until Parliament alters the law. Whether it does so will depend upon medical, social, ethical and political considerations which it is beyond the capacity of any purely legal analysis to resolve.

However, as an academic lawyer who has previously analysed

the law in remarkably similar terms to those adopted by the majority in *Gillick*[52], and as a member of a law reform agency which has twice expressed the view that to speak of parental 'rights' is misleading both as a matter of law and of ordinary language[53], it is impossible not to welcome the analysis of the parent–child relationship which may well have commended itself to the whole House. But it must also be the case that parents have at least *some* pre-emptive claims which exist unless and until the courts take them away. A parent must, for example, have the right to take a new-born baby home from hospital unless some specific and justifiable action is taken to prevent this. 'Good enough' parents must be allowed to bring up their own children in their own way, not only for their own sakes and that of their children, but also for the sake of a society which believes in individuality and freedom. The *Gillick* decision has certainly not supplied us with all the answers.

Notes and references

1 The Times, 18 October 1985.

2 [1984] QB 581, Woolf J.

3 [1985] 2 WLR 413.

4 Emergencies and parental abandonment or abuse: see page 170.

5 [1976] Fam 185.

6 442 US 584 (1979).

7 Under the 14th Amendment, '... nor shall any State deprive any person of life, liberty or property, without due process of law; nor deny any person within its jurisdiction the equal protection of the laws.'

8 There is extensive American literature on this subject. See particularly: J P Wilson. The rights of adolescents in the mental health system. Lexington, 1978; J Ellis. Volunteering children: parental commitment of minors to mental institutions. California Law Review 62, 1974, 840; Mental hospitalisation of children and the limits of parental authority. Yale Law Journal, 88, 1978, 186; L O Gostin. Current legal concepts in mental retardation in the United States: emerging constitutional issues. In: M Craft (ed) Tredgold's mental ratardation. London, Bailliere, 1979.

9 The leading discussion is: P D C Skegg. Consent to medical procedures on minors. MLR 36, 1973, 370; see also Glanville Williams. Textbook of criminal law, second edition. London, Stevens, 1983, pages 525–528; D Foulkes. Consent to medical treatment. NLJ 120, 1970, 194. For discussions of the common law before the Family Law Reform Act 1969 see H L Nathan, 1st Baron Nathan, and Barrowclough Anthony R. Medical negligence, being the law of negligence in relation to the medical profession and hospitals. London, Butterworth, 1957, chapter 7; page 176 was cited with approval in *Johnston v Wellesley Hospital*. Dominion Law Reports (3d), 17, 139 at page 145, and by the majority in *Gillick*. For a general discussion, see Lord Devlin. Medicine and the law. In: Samples of law making. Oxford, Oxford University Press, 1962.

10 J Goldstein. For Harald Lasswell: some reflections on human dignity, entrapment, informed consent and the plea bargain. Yale Law Journal 84, 1974–75, 683.

11 *Chatterton v Gerson* [1981] QB 432; *Hills v Potter* [1984] 1 WLR 641; *Sidaway v Board of Governors of Bethlem Royal Hospital and the Maudsley Hospital* [1985] 2 WLR 480.

12 See 11 above.

13 The so-called 'Bolam test' adopted in *Bolam v Friern Hospital Management Committee* 1 WLR 582.

14 *Per* Lord Bridge at page 505; Lord Keith agreed with Lord Bridge; Lord Templeman added a similar qualification – that the doctor ought to draw attention to risks which were special in kind or in magnitude or to the particular patient; Lord Diplock adopted the *Bolam* test without qualification; Lord Scarman, however, would have adopted the 'prudent patient' test – what would such a patient regard as material to his right to choose – rather than the test of what a reasonable doctor would see fit to tell him.

15 It is noteworthy that, as explained on page 165, Lord Scarman laid down quite a stringent test for a child's capacity to consent: a doctrine that consent must be truly 'informed', which he alone has propounded in English law, may have as its corollary the requirement that the patient be capable of profiting from that information: the tendency may then be to deprive people of reduced abilities, such as mentally handicapped or child patients, of the right to choose: it was this feature of the doctrine which Professor Goldstein attacked in the article cited at 10 above.

16 *R v Harling* [1938] 1 A11 ER 307; *R v Howard* [1966] 1 WLR 13.

17 Under what is now the Sexual Offences Act 1956, sections 5 and 6; the age of 16 was first adopted in the Criminal Law Amendment Act 1885.

18 *R v D* 1984 AC 778.

19 For example, beneficial contracts of employment.

20 Age of Marriage Act 1929; apparently 16 was chosen because it was by then the age of consent to sexual intercourse; intercourse between a husband and wife whose marriage is recognised as valid in English law is not 'unlawful' even if the wife is under 16: see *Mohamed v Knott* [1969] 1 QB 1.

21 See *R v Hayes*[1977] 1 WLR 234.

22 See, for example, *J M (a minor) v Runeckles* (1984) 79 Cr App R 255.

23 In *R v D* [1985] AC 778, at page 806, for example, he said 'I see no good reason why, in relation to the kidnapping of a child, it should not in all cases be the absence of the child's consent which is material, whatever its age may be.... In the case of an older child, however, it must, I think, be a question of fact for a jury whether the child concerned has sufficient understanding and intelligence to give its consent....'

24 Both their Lordships based their conclusions on the existence of the statutory offence of unlawful sexual intercourse; there is, however, some logical difficulty in holding that an *unmarried* girl under 16 is not competent to decide to practice sex and contraception, when she may be competent to contract a marriage which English law will recognise as valid, and presumably then would be competent to decide to practise sex and contraception.

25 See particularly J C Hall. The waning of parental rights. Cambridge Law Review, 1972B, 248; J M Eekelaar. What are parental rights? Law Quarterly Review, 89, 1973, 210; B M Dickens. The modern function and limits of parental rights. Law Quarterly Review, 1981, 462.

26 Section 5 of the Law Reform (Miscellaneous Provisions) Act 1970 abolished actions for deprivation of services through rape, seduction or enticement and for harbouring.

27 Section 2 of the Administration of Justice Act 1982 abolished actions for deprivation of services through torts against the child.

28 Guardianship of Minors Act 1971, section 1.

29 [1970] AC 668.

30 Children Act 1975, Part II, introduces the possibility of third parties applying for legal custody of a child in their care; other examples are the right of grandparents to apply for access to children following parental death or separation, or of stepparents to apply for custody following parental divorce: there is no universal power of application.

31 For example, in care proceedings under Children and Young Persons Act 1969, section 1.

32 Any person may apply to make a child a ward of court or, presumably, invoke the court's other inherent powers; the only recognised limitations upon the wardship jurisdiction are 1) where some competing public interest (such as freedom of expression) should take priority over the protection of the child (see *Re X* [1975] Fam 47) and 2) where it might interfere with the statutory powers of local authorities in care cases (see *A v Liverpool City council* [1982] AC 363 and *Re W (a minor) (wardship jurisdiction)* [1975] 2 WLR 892).

33 *Re D* (see 5 above); see also *Re B (a minor) (wardship medical treatment)* [1981] 1 WLR 1421.

34 Guardianship of Minors Act 1971, section 1 applies to 'any proceedings in any court' where, *inter alia*, the upbringing of a minor is in issue.

35 However, Lord Justice Eveleigh did recognise that the decision must be based upon the child's welfare: the question was who should have the burden of taking a risk.

36 Child Care Act 1980, section 3, over children already received into care under section 2 of that act.

37 Guardianship Act 1973, section 1(1).

38 Children Act 1975, section 85(1).

39 Children Act 1975, section 86.

40 See section 33(3) of the Children Act 1975 which, in defining the qualifications of third parties who may apply for legal custody, must contemplate that parents will usually have legal custody and thus, by giving consent to the application, may shorten the period for which the third party must have had care of the child before applying.

41 Sir William Blackstone. Commentaries on the laws of England, book I, first edition, 1765, page 434.

42 See 41 above, page 441.

43 See 41 above, page 440.

44 (1883) 24 Ch D 317.

45 The precise extent of parental powers and duties in respect of their children's property is open to debate: see Law Commission working paper no 91, Guardianship, 1985, paragraphs 2.32–2.34; parental powers to give or withhold consent to marriage are set out in Marriage Act 1949, section 3 and schedule 2.

46 Children and Young Persons Act 1933, section 1, especially, section 1(2)(a).

47 Education Act 1944, section 36; these duties are also laid upon people with actual care of a child, but parents may have them whether or not they have actual care.

48 [1970] 1 QB 357.

49 See 48 above, at page 372.

50 *R v Howes* (1860) 1 E & E 332; this case was much relied upon by the Court of Appeal in *Gillick* for the proposition that the age at which children acquire capacity to consent to medical treatment must be fixed and cannot depend upon their individual abilities; it was rejected by the majority in the House of Lords.

51 [1970] 1 QB 357, at page 369.

52 The argument in this paper is substantially unchanged since it was first delivered in March 1985; see also Brenda Hoggett. Mental health law, second edition. Sweet and Maxwell, 1984, pages 91–93.

53 Law Commission. Illegitimacy. Law Commission, no 118, 1982, paragraph 4.18; and Law Commission working paper no 91. Guardianship, 1985, paragraph 1.11.

EVERYDAY ETHICS: PREVENTION, PATERNALISM AND THE PILL

Roger Higgs

Ethical thought and discussion is vital for the future health of medicine and all involved in it: such a claim must lie behind the work that has gone into this volume. But where should the concentration of attention lie? What is the proper field of enquiry? With such a range of issues, such an array of acts and actors to examine, where can medical ethics make its best contribution? Two separate fields of study can be discerned. The first examines technical advance, where there is a challenge, or apparent threat, to the accepted boundaries of life or of humanity. Medical science, whether in the form of clinical treatment or research, urgently needs guidance here, with issues such as replacement surgery, gene manipulation, or embryo research. Here the sheer drama of new and exciting achievements in the high technology of specialist medicine absorbs much of our attention (as well as our finance), and creates the need for immediate solutions.[1] This is reflected in some of the contributions to this book, and rightly so.

In contrast, little public attention is paid to the ordinary issues of everyday practice, issues that concern us all, where our values and assumptions are daily put to the test in encounters between patient and professional. This might be called medical ethics' second front. Here boundaries are still an issue, and health professionals are also on the frontiers of knowledge, but it is the knowledge of their true role, concern about what patient and professional can or should do, or what society is allowing or asking each to do, that is in question. Ian Kennedy has reviewed the recent responses of the law in mediating and monitoring the relationship between patient and doctor, and pointed in particular to the Gillick case, discussed in full by Mrs Hoggett. In spite of the brilliant clarity of both these analyses, however, those working in the field of health care may lose the force of these discussions unless they are seen in context. The following discussion therefore looks further at day to day issues, from the standpoint of a practitioner.

Everyday medical ethics thus concerns itself with the perplexities and paradoxes daily presented to all patients and professionals in the medical arena, but is of especial importance to anyone who works in family or community practice. Here, lines back to the central medical powerhouses are stretched to their thinnest, there are no white coats to hide behind, and consultations lie in wait for the unwary outside McDonald's or in the Sainsbury checkout queue. In this environment, demand can so easily obscure real need. Thus, it is only by establishing and monitoring priorities that the best care can be given. Medical ethics is no exception. Each consultation challenges both patient and professional to be clear about his or her own aims and values. There are few such meetings that do not raise major questions. What are the claims of autonomy, privacy, professionalism, family ties, sexuality? Is it happiness or health, a long life, or a gay one? Should we concentrate on roles or rules, rights or relationships?

Within this hurley burley, one medical task emerges of prime importance – that of prevention, or anticipatory care.[2] If we cannot cure, we must comfort – but better still, surely, to prevent in the first place. Much has been written about how important this is to do, and even more about how difficult it is to achieve. There seems to have been little discussion, however, as to the moral issues in preventative work, and yet these have been brought into sharp relief by changes in attitudes and recent events.

Three areas

I should like to look into three areas where prevention raises ethical questions. The first is represented by that of addiction, whether socialised and accepted in the form of dependency on cigarettes, alcohol or a tranquilliser, or less accepted in the form of hard drug dependency. This could be a subject in itself, but is important because it raises basic questions about individual autonomy. The second is that of behaviour change, in situations where it appears that maladaptive patterns of living or attitudes are threatening health or happiness. It is a plain across which armies of counsellors, psychologists, drug company salesmen, and alternative medicine practitioners wheel and parade with enthusiasm, often raising more dust and noise than making easily proven advances. Be that as it may, lives can be altered and unhappiness prevented, and the health workers' role in this needs to be examined, if only because, yet again, there are issues of priority at stake.

The third area is where a teenager presents for contraception. Ever since the startling case 14 years ago where the General Medical Council[3] upheld the decision of a doctor to divulge a teenager's family planning secrets to the girl's father, medical practice and medical establishment rulings in this country appear to have become more and more liberal – almost as if in penance for the naked old fashioned paternalism, symbolic, moral and actual, that this GMC ruling represented. Doctors were persuaded that prevention of pregnancy as well as disease was their task, and uneasily moved towards the suggestion underlined by a DHSS circular and supported by a new GMC, that it was both permissible and important for a doctor to provide family planning for a young woman, even under 16, and even when she could not be persuaded to allow discussion with the parents. This was abruptly halted by the Appeal judgement in the Gillick case, and although the final decision in the Lords has gone some way to reverse this, the challenge both to the medical role and to teenagers' autonomy in society remains.

Five cases

Five recent consultations illustrate these three difficult areas.

The first was reported second hand from a young colleague who is a heavy smoker, and after a long consultation with his own doctor was still furious that the doctor was not immediately prepared to give him 'something to stop him smoking' straight away. He felt it was the doctor's job to take on his bad habit, and to stop it.

The second was dramatically presented on the recent Doctors' Dilemmas series on BBC2 TV. A young wife wants a new life without further children, and so seeks family planning from her doctor in total confidence. The young husband, however, wants more children, perhaps specifically a son, and comes to the doctor to ask for help, thinking that he is infertile but not knowing that his wife is using contraception. The doctor in front of 3.5 million viewers or so, struggles in an unsatisfactory but probably well meaning way to sort this out, and in so doing finds himself having to tell lies to both husband and wife, and thus pleases neither the couple nor the panel of commentators later in the programme. What these commentaries seemed to miss was the doctor's ill-expressed feeling that he should, in some way, be preventing disaster within this family by maintaining contact with them. Continuity of care, something that most family doctors feel they should be offering to their patients, was delineated by the commentators merely as a power game. While not in any way enjoying the deception into which that doctor was drawn, I think this case highlights important facets of the doctor–patient relationship concerning prevention and the contract.

The last three consultations bring us to an area on which I wish to concentrate. In the week on which the appeal court ruled on Mrs Gillick's case against the DHSS notice on contraception for minors[4], three consultations that were pertinent presented:

> Denise, nearly 16, was living with her boyfriend and his parents in a stable relationship. She was not in contact with her own parents now, but was working towards re-establishing it. However, she had wanted and had received contraceptive advice and help over the previous six months, which now appeared difficult to continue.

> Anne, aged $14\frac{1}{2}$, came to consult about abdominal pain, and in the course of the consultation revealed that she had a steady relationship with a sixteen year old boy, using amazing and primitive methods of birth control that would normally be considered highly unreliable. She wanted to use the pill, but refused to tell her parents and preferred to go back to her former unreliable methods.

Lastly, Mary, a woman of 26, in the course of discussion about how her marriage was not working out, revealed haltingly that as an early teenager she had been regularly interfered with by her uncle, who was also her guardian, with the connivance of her aunt. Years later, she still found it hard to forget and forgive, mostly herself.

The appeal court ruling on the Gillick case offered the doctor three choices if a woman under 16 wanted contraception and would not consult her parents: refusing to help, claiming that the case was an emergency, or applying to court. Both Anne and Denise could be expected to return, while still schoolchildren, with an unwanted pregnancy. Emergency is a hard word to define, in theory and in practice, and recourse to court would be quite inappropriate in these cases, as in most. Mary raised a different issue, but might have come to see her doctor, as a way into the problem, for contraception when she was younger.

While the decision of the House of Lords has now clarified this and allows the doctor to respond under the DHSS guidelines (see Brenda Hoggett's chapter, p 158) many people remain sympathetic to the thinking behind the appeal court decision. In particular, relief has been expressed that at last public figures have spoken out to prevent what appears to some to be an 'epidemic' of early teenage sex. This misunderstanding should be cleared before we move on. Evidence from a number of sources suggests that most teenagers attending for family planning have already made up their minds about their sexual intentions or have already started having intercourse. Some may come to prepare themselves before entering a relationship. By and large, however, though numbers are few – and many young women are brought by their parents anyway – those approaching doctors for contraceptives are not virgins. Thus we should look clearly at the issue, which is not about the prevention of teenage sex, but the prevention of unwanted pregnancy.

Preventive medicine

Before we go further into this specific area, let us consider some of the general issues of prevention or anticipatory care. Although this is a long way back in the drawer and can get hidden under all sorts of apparently more urgent tasks, most doctors and nurses would agree that it is one of the tasks in medicine that is most worthwhile. Some go further and would suggest that a failure to benefit others when in a position to do so violates a professional duty. Certainly, looking into history, preventive medicine is now recognised as one of the medals among the honours heaped by later generations on Victorian health workers. Even for railway enthusiasts, that was the age of the drain. Some of the stories are symbolic. The method of spread of cholera was first both confirmed and the disease prevented at a single blow in Soho, when John Snow, anaesthetist and general practitioner, noted that all his cholera cases seemed to be clustered round one pump.[5] At that time the idea that germs could be waterborne was novel. Snow had thought this out carefully, and removed the pump handle. Cholera in his district stopped. Case proved, disease prevented. The pub in Broadwick Street still commemorates the event and the people he saved. Today we do not have quite such simple models in our major killer diseases. However, whether it is lung cancer or heart attacks, alcohol or child abuse, road accidents, suicides, or AIDS, most modern epidemics have at least one major preventable element that can be efficiently and effectively pursued by doctors and patients together.

When it comes to public policy, it is hard not to be persuaded of the worth of spending some time and effort now to improve health and save money later, even though it is difficult to analyse the costs and benefits of many preventative schemes in a way which seems realistic. Likewise, it appears to have been widely accepted that living in a complex modern society confers on the state the right or even duty to promote such programmes as immunisation or cervical screening, and to compel such measures as the wearing of car seat belts. There is little consistency in the way that different societies apply these rulings, however. Gulliver would be amused to travel between a state where drink is prohibited but everyone may carry a gun, and another where an individual may freely drink and smoke himself to death, yet be cared for in his final illness from the taxes raised in part from his more abstemious peers.

Provided effective action could be taken, these arguments suggest that the state, the professions and patients alike should in theory welcome any measures to promote health or prevent deterioration. On the 'apple a day' principle, keeping the doctor away must be considered a major social good. In practice, people are not so keen on the idea, particularly when it is applied to themselves rather than to their cohorts next door. In studies of smokers with arterial disease of the legs (which is rare in non-smokers) many sufferers, offered the choice of stopping smoking or having major reconstructive surgery of their lower limb arteries, chose the latter. Studies of a treatment of raised blood pressure which is an effective method of preventing stroke, but at some cost, show that half of those with raised pressure go undetected, only half of the detected are treated, and only half of those treated are treated effectively.[6] Whoever is primarily at fault here, to the outsider it looks suspiciously like collusion. The defence of inaction may be that the doctor is exceeding his brief by intruding into areas where a patient may not have perceived a need or requested help; or that patients have every right to drop out of a treatment programme that does not treat something we would normally call an illness, that can only be proved to be working by the person stopping the treatment and coming to grief, and that turns the well person into a patient who feels less well. No wonder, you may say, that the Chinese paid their doctors on a different system.

Contract and whole person care

If this muddle is based on an agreement, it is hard to see what form this agreement takes when it comes to the relationship between doctor and patient. Preventive care, in its broadest sense, does not quite fit in with those modern views which see this relationship as *entirely* a contract, whether the emphasis is on the narrower legal or the broader social sense of the word. The smoker, the stressed executive, the unhappy child, the grieving widow – wherever a person is, in a professional view, at risk and should be steered away from that risk, a doctor or nurse may feel that he or she should initiate activity *unrequested*. This is one factor that may distinguish what Halmos[7] calls the 'personal service professions' (medical workers, clergy, teachers, social workers) from the 'impersonal service professions' – that their 'principle function is to bring about change in the body or personality of the client'. This activity is often proactive, not reactive, within the context of the relationship. Thus the doctor is not just the *agent* of the patient, and the narrow view of contract does not seem enough to cover what modern, nonpaternalistic care would like to offer, or receive. Here I follow William F May[8], writing in Hastings Centre Report in 1975, who suggests that the word 'covenant' is a better expression than contract. Although 'first cousins' and similar in so many ways, in spirit or approach these words portray differences. Contracts make precise the terms of the relationship, and if these are fulfilled obligation under contract is discharged, and that is the end of the matter. But covenants have 'a gratuitous, growing edge to them that nourishes rather than limits relationships' and may outline communal rather than bipolar relationships. Be that as it may, the agreement between doctor and patient contains some sort of promise that guards against minimalism, and offers the prospect of flexible, intelligent and skillful anticipation and interpretation to preserve individual health. Within this partnership (see page 000), 'anticipatory care' may be a better term than prevention as it gives a more realistic view of what can or cannot be done.

Expectations may be even more difficult to evaluate when it comes to a relationship which emphasises the holistic or 'whole person' approach. It is hard not to catch the irony in many official pronouncements about this issue. The World Health Organization set the appropriate universalist phrase in their charter. 'Health is a state of complete mental and social well-being and not merely the absence of disease or infirmity.' Seen, as we have said elsewhere, as a goal for the *patient* this is useful, but as a trades description for health professionals it would probably cause a walkout. Nevertheless, it is what most enlightened family doctors would take as the ideal definition in a far from ideal world. In spite of the fragmentation and ambivalence of much that a primary care worker lives or deals with, whole person medicine is not what it is sometimes seen as – an alternative; it is an essential, the essence of proper professional care. So often the term is applied to new alternative treatments which lie outside orthodox medicine, expressed only by those with a yen for yin and yang. But whole person medicine involves something much deeper and more important – a radical change of perspective on the part of both patient and therapist, to take positive health as the goal. At this point enters the classical question about the Californian psychiatrists – how many are needed to change a lightbulb? The answer, of course, is only one, but the lightbulb must *really* want to change. However we express ideas of prevention and anticipatory care whether using a medicalised view, with words like 'compliance', or a person-centred approach, no change is possible without the involvement of the patient's will in the task as well as his or her acquiescence. Thus, the impact of whole person medicine is clear. It is a business of *sharing* between patient and therapist, the goals agreed, each his or her own person, autonomous.

The concept of autonomy has been hovering behind much of what has been discussed so far. Self governance, having the freedom to make one's own individual choices, 'being one's own person' – all are implied by what has been said so far if any preventive measure is to be effective. Far from challenging personal autonomy, as often so many feel that preventive measures seem to do, they either cannot operate outside the context of autonomy, or else they enhance it. In the normal conditions of western society, whatever the state may decree, unless the lightbulb is intent on change, mega-jacuzzi-loads of Californian psychiatrists are ineffective.

Doubts may creep in, however, if we return to our cases. What about the smoker? He seems autonomous, yet Kant, concerned about the moral autonomy of the *will* (as opposed to Mill's individuality of thought and action)[9] might well have regarded his actions constrained so completely by desire and habit as to be definitely heteronomous. Certainly someone on heavier drugs would seem to most of us to have compromised his or her free status. So perhaps my friend was justified in his annoyance, on grounds of morality and professionalism as well as politeness, at his shoulder-shrugging brush off. Some might claim that more active involvement by the doctor is needed to come to the patient's aid, a paternalistic shove to push his moral autonomy count back to nearer what it should be. Those in thrall often excite in their therapists a liberating zeal which paradoxically requires major paternalistic actions or attitudes for success – the phrases of revolutionary politics echoing in the area of medical ethics. However, most people would prefer to follow a liberal rather than liberating path, and 'allow' the addict to declare his best intentions in a symbolic if short-lived statement before a paternalistic programme is introduced.

The husband seeking a child was likewise not in a position of free choice, because he was not in full possession of the available facts, being kept on the end of a string (or even a coil) by his wife, more a con trick than a contract. The enormity of such marital games may be unusual, but the prevalence is not. By colluding and manipulating, the doctor drew the patient further into the toils, reduced his autonomy, and made him sicker (and the doctor compromised his own autonomy into the bargain). This process of temporarily reducing autonomy by creating dependence is part of many therapeutic regimes, but in this case it was based on deception and therefore seems doubly dubious. Detecting the moral lesion may have helped the doctor to put responsibility for action back where it belonged, with the couple. This case also makes us realise that autonomy has its physical as well as conceptual limits. No man is an island, and no one fully autonomous. A cynical bachelor might well say that all married people have diminished autonomy, and are therefore morally sick, but then that is a particular view!

Two important threads should be drawn out of this. One is that our thinking about freedom of action in a medical context should not be trapped, as the thinking of 'high tech' organ-based medical specialities often is, into conceptualising the body as *containing* all conditions. Interpretative sociology, life – events work, anthropology have all shown us that symptoms in a person may be symbols of what happens outside that person, or a reflection of the environment. It may thus be the surroundings and not the internal milieu that requires the study or creates the challenge for therapy. Freedom of choice is 'within which' or 'between'; autonomy is *contextual*. To put it another way, being autonomous is in some senses a transitive, not intransitive expression and requires us to say more. People are autonomous *with respect* to something. Like a musical chord, autonomy demands to be put into a key, each of which, as musicologists inform us, may have a specific meaning different from the others. Sexuality may be one of these 'keys' or contexts which both complicates and clarifies our understanding of teenagers' developing independence.

Thus we reach the teenager who approaches the practitioner for contraception. How autonomous is she? One answer would be that she is compromised by virtue of being a child, and even if one thinks of autonomy as a sliding scale (or a slippery slope) she has not yet reached the stage of full allowable self-governance where such a choice can be morally allowable. Mrs Hoggett has clarified some of the confusing aspects of British law in this respect, but there remain the views of society and her family as to her true status, which influences the style of covenant or partnership that can arise between her and her doctors. She may be a child with respect to life assurance or knowing how to work a word processor, but by presenting for contraception she has defined herself as already having made a responsible 'adult' decision. This could be claimed partly because, as I have said, her decision to have sex nearly always predates the request for contraception, and because sex in this context is biologically an adult and not an infantile activity. Finally it could be claimed because of the very maturity of that request in itself. It seems very odd that in spite of this we should cast doubts on her autonomous capacity to consent. Before we can take this issue further, however, to look at the rights of parents or children, we should examine, in summary, the convergence of professional ideas about prevention and patients' views of autonomy in these cases.

Thus, sickness may reduce autonomy by making the patient necessarily dependent on nurse or physician. I have argued elsewhere that autonomy is a sign of health, in the sense that health is only restored when the patient is as fully able to make choices as he or she ever was before the illness. There are thus arguments for paternalism in some form in emergency medicine, and it is hard to see how paternalism, in some shape, strong or weak, could ever be banished from hospital wards, even if there was a patient advocate attached by string to every bed chart.

However, in the issue of prevention, the matter is somewhat different. Here we are presupposing a relatively well individual, who may be informed of the risks he or she is running, may discuss them, and may make sober decisions about them untrammelled by dependence on ministering angels, clinical tubes or cold bedpans. Given such circumstances, in spite of the best descriptions and most eloquent persuasions many adults fail to take advice or avoiding action.

The reasons for this apparent failure are complex, and are possibly related to the individual's views of risk, or different perceptual sets of cultural values. It remains that many fail to comply with the suggestions. But seen against this background of worthwhile, objectively and professionally approved preventive action failing to move *adults*, we come to a contrast. The adolescent seeking family planning comes not as a patient with a sickness nor with a condition that is a precursor of sickness. She does not even have to be cajoled into attendance. She is well, autonomous within the context of her request, complies instantly, in fact so instantly that it is she who requests the general measures to be adopted, not the physician.

She is not ill, she has no compromised autonomy, she does not have a premorbid condition, she does not need to be persuaded to comply; she just turns up saying 'Please, I want contraception. Now. For very good reasons. To prevent a disaster. Just don't tell my mum. Haven't I got the right?'

What are children's rights?

However unsatisfactory the current usage of 'rights' language may be, and however much we should prefer to examine the concept of duties, the question of the rights of minors urgently needs attention. The classical statement is the Declaration of Rights of the Child by the United Nations in 1959. This outlines a series of ten principles concerned with the welfare of children. Of particular interest is the ninth principle, which covers protection against all forms of neglect, cruelty and exploitation. This principle follows the more general statement, that we should be offering the child special protection, opportunities and facilities to enable him or her to develop in a healthy manner, in conditions of freedom and dignity: the best interests of the child to be of paramount consideration. The increasing understanding of the threat to life, health and happiness of some children, given stark reality by a number of publicised tragic deaths from non-accidental injury in this country, has made us concentrate more and more on the aspect of *protection from harm*. The child is weak and vulnerable, and the state's resources must be mobilised in protection, 'the best interests of the child to be of paramount consideration'. But, who is to decide the best interests of the child, and how can harm be quantified and balanced?

In approaching the first question, society would normally leave this decision to the parents, if their decision was wise. As Mrs Hoggett has explained, the law has followed society's view that parents are not the final arbiters, and they may have dwindling authority and reduced responsibilities as the child gets older. When children are young, health visitors and social workers in particular have special responsibilities to prevent physical harm, and may be subjected to trial by media if they misjudge the gravity of the situation. Educational authorities are also given limited powers to intervene if a child is being deprived of proper tuition. In both instances the child may not ask for protection, but it seems particularly perverse that in medical care the child who wisely requests it should be effectively denied it. Thus, doctors do have an important stake in this delicate area, not as some unpleasant agent for state eugenics or family dispersal, as seemed to be suggested in part of the Gillick trial, and certainly not without regard to other risks facing the child, but because the child requests it, and doctors have a duty to care, and, where appropriate, to protect. It may be no protection for the child if the doctor refuses to do what the parents request against the child's wishes (see Brenda Hoggett's chapter, p 158) since determined and less scrupulous adults may find a professional who, this time, agrees with them.

Thus while the rights of the child to protection have become more important, another movement has been growing. This sees the rights which are most under threat to be those relating to the right of the child to be treated *as a person*. They include the right to individual freedom and self-determination, to be treated in the same way as an adult, as having legitimate desires, free choice, and the responsibility to make that choice. The contrast between welfare rights and rights as an individual often seems to be a debate between what the child needs and what the child wants or, put succinctly, between protecting children and protecting their rights. In writings by people like Holt and Farson[10], the children's rights movement can sound extreme – including demands for political power and things which adults have yet to achieve. Some might feel the need to give every child a childhood, but not yet an adulthood.

Nevertheless the child has growing rights of free choice as well as welfare rights, and the right to society's protection. The famous Section 18 of the Child Care Act (1980) rolls the two neatly (but perhaps confusingly) into one. Professionals must give first consideration to the welfare of the child in their care, must ascertain and give due consideration to the child's wishes and feelings: since presumably children not in care must be treated in a similar way, these rights impose on society particular duties – in this case, the twin duties to protect and to give due consideration to the child's wishes and feelings. If the child seeks protection from pregnancy and wishes for it, it is hard to see how anyone on this basis could refuse to provide protection. If the child understands what is involved, has the capacity to make the decision, and the decision is wise, those in positions of trust with children or teenagers are left with the emphasis not on rights but a clear duty – to protect the child from harm. Here the prime duties of parents and doctors totally coincide, provided that a clear concept is obtained of the harmful issues involved.

But what is most harmful to the teenager still under parental care? I have discussed elsewhere[11] how the very objective sound to the word 'harm' conceals many of its subjective features. There are hierarchies and dimensions within this word which can create considerable disagreement between individuals viewing it from different personal or role perspectives. To balance these views requires openness and care. The parent may attach real importance to the loss of childhood innocence, physical and psychological, involved in early sexual experiences, the destruction of family trust, and the potential threat to physical health of the teenager (such as venereal disease, long-term risk of cervical cancer, side effects of contraception). The child may be under pressure to act in an uncharacteristic way, or even against her will, by her peers. The doctor or nurse may be concerned by these divergent opinions but may also place greater emphasis on the harm of not providing contraception: an unwanted pregnancy, more risky in an early teenager, and the guilt or disturbance of the experience. They may worry about the possibility of the teenager resorting to 'backstreet' abortion, concealing the pregnancy and requesting a termination later, or having an unsupervised pregnancy and a concealed birth. There may be concern over the health of a young family – its stability, the quality of the mother–child relationship, and the limited horizons that this creates for the young mother. The diminution of trust is an issue here as it is with the parents, but with the added risk that should there be incest or other problems in the family there is no easy way for the teenager to approach her doctor unless she can receive an open reception with totally confidential guidance. If parents and doctors have a duty to protect adolescent children from harm, that means that they should allow the adolescents, when family processes fail, to protect themselves.

Adults know too little about teenagers' lives – and perhaps that is how teenagers in every era wish it to remain! Where there is real conflict and risk of harm, both parents and teenager may need help, and help should be obtained from a source which everyone can trust. Recourse to law is too cumbersome for this delicate area, and of necessity makes public what should decently be kept private – there can be few who would welcome a discussion of their personal sexual feelings and actions in court, even anonymously. Processes must be used which preserve privacy, trust, and amour propre, and which allow for growth of understanding, rather than antipathy, between everyone concerned. For many years society has allowed doctors and others working in health care to provide help in the privacy of a consultation. Other agencies at school or in youth services have a part to play also, but teenagers must never be deprived of the opportunity to share a problem in confidence with an appropriate professional.

In that confidential discussion the legal principles outlined by the House of Lords in the Gillick case will for the moment provide guidelines. But more may be required. Everyday ethics require an up to the minute 'on your toes' response in which the relevant principles can be balanced and analysed with due regard for the autonomy of those involved, for issues of benefit and harm in prevention, and for rights and duties. The decisions reached will need to take account of many other factors – family and societal responsibilities, religious conviction, professional obligations, medical risks. Help must be provided which obtains a proper balance of rights and responsibilities for the best interest of the young person.

No matter what is needed in the care of teenagers, in general the question of prevention remains a prime duty of doctors, to be brought about by enhanced relationship with patients that is more than a simple contractual one. The morality of everyday practice requires a method of approach that can scrutinise these relationships and use emotional as well as rational understanding to examine values as well as facts. This will in turn require a type of double perspective, an empathetic attempt to see from the viewpoint of patient and relative as well as professional. Medical ethics has been made for man, not man for medical ethics, and high technology in the medical, legal or philosophical sense is not what is needed here. Our responses should be rooted in everyday life.

Notes and references

1 This article is based on a lecture given at King's College London on 25 February 1985 entitled 'The Hi-Tech Hi-Jack: must medical ethics go the same way?' Parts of it are also derived from the National Children's Home Convocation Lecture (1984) 'Medical and Social Work Ethics', NCH occasional paper no 6.

2 This has been studied in primary care in a series of Royal College of General Practitioners (London) publications:
Royal College of General Practitioners. Promoting prevention. London, RCGP, 1983. (RCGP occasional paper 22).
Royal College of General Practitioners. Health and prevention in primary care: report of a working party appointed by the Council of the Royal College of General Practitioners (Chairman: John Horder) London, RCGP, 1981. (Report from general practice 18).
Royal College of General Practitioners. Prevention of arterial disease in general practice: report of a sub-committee of the Royal College of General Practitioners' working party on prevention (Chairman: Julian Tudor Hart) London, RCGP, 1981. (Report from general practice 19).

Royal College of General Practitioners. Prevention of psychiatric disorders in general practice: report of a sub-committee of the Royal College of General Practitioners' working party on prevention (Chairman: Philip Graham) London, RCGP, 1981. (Report from general practice 20).
Royal College of General Practitioners. Family planning: an exercise in preventive medicine: report of a sub-committee of the Royal College of General Practitioners' working party on prevention. London, RCGP, 1981. (Report from general practice 21).

3 Quoted in: R M Veatch. A theory of medical ethics. New York, Basic Books, 1981, pages 141–149.

4 *Gillick v West Norfolk and Wisbech Area Health Authority and Another* before Lords Justice Everleigh, Fox and Parker: Law Report, The Times, 21 December 1984, page 9.

5 In 1855 Snow wrote a book entitled On the mode of communication of cholera.

6 J Tudor Hart. Hypertension. Edinburgh, Churchill Livingstone, 1980; and ABC of hypertension, British Medical Association, 1981.

7 P Halmos. The personal service society. Constable, 1970, page 22.

8 W F May. Code and covenant or philanthropy and contract? Hastings Centre report, vol 5, December 1975: 29–38.

9 See T L Beauchamp and J E Childress. Principles of biomedical ethics. Oxford, Oxford University Press, 1983, pages 59–64.

10 This is reviewed well in: M D A Freeman. The rights and wrongs of children. London, Frances Pinter, 1983.

11 A Campbell and R Higgs. In that case. London, Darton Longman and Todd, 1982, pages 85–89.

INDEX

abortion: and Jewish medical ethics 123–4; legal cases 9
Abortion Act (1967) 97
addiction, treatment 178–9, 185
Administration of Justice Act (1982) 166
age: and consent 163–4; of discretion 169
anticipatory care *see* preventive medicine
Aristotle 72
artificial insemination by donor (AID) 80, 86–7, 124–5
autonomy, and preventive medicine 185–8

Bailey, Leonard 24
Bayles, Michael 143
Begotten or Made? (O'Donovan) 29, 30, 54
behaviour change, ethical questions 179, 180
Ben Gurion University, Centre for Jewish Medical Ethics 117
Bible, and Jewish medical ethics 115–16, 118
Bioethics and Belief (Mahoney) 33
biological gradient 132–3
Blackstone, Sir William, *Commentaries* on the laws of England 167–8

Brandon, Lord 158, 164
British Medical Association, *Handbook of Medical Ethics* 11

Campbell, C A 67
Catholic bishops: and the soul 72–3, 74; and Warnock Committee 29, 40–1
Child Care Act (1980) 190
children: consent 162–5, 165–6; and High Court powers 166–7; medical treatment, and parents 158–61, 170; and parental rights 165–71; psychiatric treatment 159–60; rights 161–5, 187, 188–92
Children Act (1975) 167
cholera, cause 135–6, 182
Christianity, and personhood 71–3
Clarkson, C M V 141
community medicine 127, 136, 178
compensation, monetary 19
conception, artificially-assisted *see in vitro* fertilisation
confidentiality 17–18
consent 12, 14; children's 162–5, 165–6; informed 13, 162; legal cases 9, 12–15, 162; real 162–3
context, importance of 30

194

contraception: conflict of interests 180; provision to young girls 9, 15–16, 158, 171, 179, 180–1, 187, 190–1
Cotton, Baby 82, 84, 85
Cotton, Kim 82
crime, as symptom of social disorder 152
criminal law, and responsibility 139–55
criminal liability, moral basis 140–5
cyclosporin 24

Data Protection Act (1984) 18
death: definition 24; *see also* mortality
Denning, Lord 169
Diplock, Lord 14
doctor–patient relationship: and children 15–16, 189; contract 183–4, 192; definition 9–11, 13, 15–16; truth-telling in 118–19, 180, 186; whole person care 184–5
doctors: accountability 19–20; children, medical treatment of 160–1, 164–5, 167, 170, 171; conflict of loyalties 14–15, 180, 186; contraception, provision to young girls 9, 15–16, 158, 171, 179, 180–1, 187, 188, 190–1; and everyday ethical questions 178; and legal responsibility 139, 145–8, 150–1, 154–5; preventive medicine 178–9, 182–3; smoking habits 130–1; and unemployment 136
Doctors' Dilemmas, television series 180
Doll, R 130, 132
donors, heart transplant, care of 23, 24
donors, in IVF 42–3

drug dependency, treatment 178–9, 185
Dunstan, Gordon 33, 38

Edwards, R G 38
embryos: research on 28, 31–4, 43–4, 45–7, 77; soul 72–4; status 32, 33, 74–6; *see also* foetus
employment, benefits of 134
epidemiology 127
epilepsy, as legal defence 148–9, 151–2
ethics *see* medical ethics
euthanasia, and Jewish medical ethics 119–22
Evans, D W 24
experimentation 24, 26–7, 28; on embryos 31–4, 43–4, 45–7, 77; hazardous 122

Fae, Baby 24, 25, 26
Fagin, L 133
Family Law Reform Act (1969) 163–4, 166
family planning *see* contraception
family practitioners *see* doctors
fertilisation: artificially-induced *see* *in vitro* fertilisation; trans-species 45–6
foetus, potential personhood 63, 64–8
Fox, A J 131, 132
Fraser, Lord 163, 165, 171
Frey, A G 59

General Medical Council 179; and incompetence 20–1; *Professional Conduct and Discipline* 'blue book' 11
Gillick, Victoria 15–16, 17, 18, 158; *see also* legal cases

Harefield Hospital, heart transplants 24

harm, differing views of 190–1
Hart, H L A 140–1, 142, 147, 150, 152
health: holistic approach 184–5; and smoking 130–1; and social class 131; and unemployment 127–36
heart transplants: benefit 23, 24; donors, care of 23, 24; infant 22, 24–7; resources 23, 24
Hill, A B 130, 132
Hoggett, Brenda 15, 38, 178, 187, 189
Homicide Act (1957) 139
homosexual couples, and IVF 31, 41
human being, definition 55–6, 77
human life: beginning point 55–6, 123; distinctive features 58–9, 61–2; value 56–8, 59; *see also* life; personhood
Human Fertilisation and Embryology, Committee of Enquiry, Report *see* Warnock report
Human Procreation: Ethical Aspects of the New Techniques (Council for Science and Society) 30, 33

identity, in Jewish medical ethics 124
incompetence, doctors' 19–21
infertility: increasing 80; treatment for 80; *see also in vitro* fertilisation
information, protection of 18
in vitro fertilisation (IVF) 22; donors 42–3; eligibility for 41–2; objections to 28–34; supervisory body 48–50

Jacobovits, Sir Immanuel 55–6
Jahoda, M 134
Jewish law, and medical ethics 116–17
Jewish medical ethics: origins 115–17
Jones, D R 131, 132
judicial law 7–8, 9

Kant, Immanuel 185
Keating, H M 141
Kennedy, Ian 38, 177
Kohlberg, L 67
Kreitman, N 127–8, 133

Latey, Mr Justice 82
law, the: and developments in medical science 7–9; and responsibility 139–55
Law Reform (Miscellaneous Provisions) Act (1970) 166
legal cases:
Emeh v Kensington and Chelsea and Westminster Area Health Authority (1984) 9
Freeman v Home Office (1984) 14–15, 17
Gillick v West Norfolk and Wisbech Area Health Authority (1985) 9, 15–16, 17–18, 47–8, 158, 161, 162–5, 166–72, 179, 180, 181
Hewer v Bryant (1970) 168–9
In re B (a minor) (1981) 9
J v C (1970) 166
McKay v Essex Area Health Authority (1982) 9
Parham v JR 159
Re D (a minor) (wardship: sterilisation (1976)) 159, 161
Re Agar-Ellis (1883) 168, 169
R v Arthur (1981) 9
R v D (1985) 164

R v Sullivan (1983) 138–9, 151–2
R v Sutcliffe (1981) 145–6, 148, 149, 151, 152, 154
Royal College of Nursing v DHSS (1981) 9
Sidaway v Board of Governors of the Bethlem Royal Hospital and the Maudsley Hospital (1985) 9, 12–14, 16, 47, 162
lesbian couples, and IVF 31
life: beginning point 55–6, 123; worth of 56–8, 59, 120–2, 123–4; wrongful 9, 98
litigation, increase in 9, 11
Little, M 133
Loma Linda Medical Center (Cal) 24

Mahoney, John 29–30, 33, 38
Maimonides 116, 117
malpractice litigation 18–21
May, William F 184
medical ethics: everyday issues 177–8, 191–2; and technological advance 22, 177
medical law, development of 7–9
medical science, proper goals 30–1, 34
medical technology, advances in 22–3, 177
mens rea 139, 140, 141, 142, 143, 154
mental disorder, in children 159–60
Mental Health Act (1983) 161, 163
Mill, John Stuart 185
minors *see* children
mortality: and resources 134; and unemployment 128–30, 136
Moser, K A 131, 132

National Health Service (NHS), resources 22–3

National Insurance Act (1911) 136

occupational medicine 14–15, 17
O'Donovan, Oliver 29, 54
Oliver, Michael 25
OPCS, mortality study 128–30
Opren, drug 9
Order of Christian Unity 34

Papworth Hospital, heart transplants 24
parents: and children's consent 165–6; and children's medical treatment 158–61, 170; and children's rights 161, 189; duties 168, 170; rights 16, 165–71, 172
partnership, doctor–patient 13, 14; *see also* doctor–patient relationship
paternalism: and addiction 185–6; and emergency medicine 187; and preventive medicine 187–8
patients: autonomy 185–8; definition 15; 'reasonable' 14; *see also* doctor–patient relationship
personhood: beginning point 71–4; differing views of 69–71; distinctive features 58–9, 60, 61–2, 63–4, 69; potential 62–3, 64–8; and value 60–1, 64
Platt, S 127–8, 133
potential personhood 62–3, 64–8
Powell, Enoch 27, 29, 32
power, in doctor–patient relationship 14–15, 16, 17
Practical Ethics (Singer) 54
pregnancy, prevention of 179; *see also* contraception

preventive medicine 181–3, 192; ethical questions 178–81; intervention, unsolicited 183–4; patient's autonomy 185–8
prisoners, medical treatment, consent to 14–15
privacy *see* confidentiality

'reasonable patient' test 14
reproduction, artificial aids 27, 28; *see also in vitro* fertilisation
research, medical *see* experimentation
resources, and mortality 134
responsibility: capacity conception of 153–5; character conception of 143–5, 149–50, 152–3, 154–5; and criminal liability 140–5; differing concepts of 139–40, 143–4, 154; legal concept of 139–40; philosophical concept 139
rights: after birth 55; children's 161–5, 187, 188–92; parents' 16, 165–71, 172
Roffey, Hollie 24, 25–6

Sachs, Lord Justice 168–9
Scarman, Lord 14, 65
selective treatment, legal cases 9
Singer, Peter 54
smoking: and ill health 130–1, 132; medical treatment for 179, 185
Snow, John 135–6, 182
social class and health 131
soul, formation of 72–3, 74
Steptoe, P C 38
sterilisation, failed 9
suicide and unemployment 127–8

Surrogacy Arrangements Bill (1985) 82, 103
surrogate motherhood 27, 29, 81–2; agencies 85, 93, 105–6; arguments against 84–104; child, care for 110–11; child, harming 94–9, 103; child, as product 101, 108; commercial, prohibition 105–9; as constructive abandonment 99–101, 108; and criminal law 85, 87, 93; as disposition of bodily organ 90–1, 103; as employment 89–90; as exploitation 88–9, 103; family life, abnormal 94–5, 97; financial aspects 88–94, 96, 103, 106–7, 108, 109; intermediaries 105–6, 109–10; licensing and regulation 104–5; and marital relationship 86–8, 107; means and ends 101–2, 103, 108; mother, harming 88–92; mother, role 106–9; parent–child relations 99–102; private arrangement 87–8, 93–4, 107; prohibition, total 104; public opinion on 84–6; three-parent family 86–8; women as machines 92
Surrogate Parenting Centre of Great Britain 82

Talmud, and Jewish medical ethics 116, 123
teenagers, status 187; *see also* children
Teichmann, Jenny 76
Templeman, Lord 158, 164–5, 170
Thomas Aquinas, St 72
truth, suppressing 118–19, 180, 186

Unborn Children (Protection) Bill   27, 29, 32
unemployment: female   132; and future health   133–4; and health   127–36; ill-health as cause   133–4; length of   133; and para-suicides   127–8; and social class   131
United Nations, Declaration of the Rights of the Child (1959)   188
United States: children, unwanted treatment of 159–60; President's Commission for the Study of Ethical Problems in Medicine and Biomedical and Behavioral Research 49–50; surrogacy in   81–2

value of life   120–2, 123
Warnock report (1984)   27, 28–9, 37, 48, 53, 54, 55, 77, 78; and AID   124–5; committee members   37–8; and context   30; and donors 42–3; and eligibility for treatment   41–2; embryo, status   32, 43; evidence presented   39–40; experimentation on embryos   43–4, 45–7; and infertility   40–1; morality and law   44–5; and supervisory body   48–50; surrogate motherhood   82, 83–94, 103, 105–6, 111–12; trans-species fertilisation   45–6; utilitarianism in   44–5
whooping cough vaccine   9
Winston, R   38
women, and unemployment 132
World Health Organization, Charter   184
Wootton, Baroness   152

Yacoub, Magdi   24, 25–6, 27
Yorkshire Ripper case, *R v Sutcliffe* (1981)   145–6, 148, 149, 151, 152, 154